Praise for Exit Strategies

"Such an accessible and helpful book, written with warm, meaningful and relatable experiences of "what really matters" care. Included are excellent resources and tools that we all can benefit from so that we can both help ourselves and others."

—Jennie Chin Hansen, Past CEO of the American Geriatrics Society; past President of the AARP

"This book turns a confusing, scary, and exhausting time before a death into a process that is human, manageable, and warm. And funny! Not only regular people, but also clinicians can gain a lot from reading this."

—Diane E. Meier, MD, Founder of the Center to Advance Palliative Care; Professor of Geriatrics and Palliative Medicine at the Icahn School of Medicine at Mount Sinai Hospital; past MacArthur Fellowship "Genius Grant" awardee.

"Exit Strategies is a tribute to the resilience of the human spirit, reminding us that even in our final moments, there is much to learn, laugh about, and treasure. Pan's core message is powerful: even when life is nearing its end, it still holds immense value."

—Eric Widera, M.D. Professor of Clinical Medicine, Division of Geriatrics, UCSF; Director, Hospice & Palliative Care, SFVAMC Office; Blog/Podcast: www.geripal.org

"*Exit Strategies* is must-read! Dr. Pan's honesty, wisdom and humor shed much needed light on how to navigate the end of life with grace and compassion."

—Warren Racusin Esq, chair, trusts and estates group, Lowenstein Sandler, and producer of trusts and estates podcast "Splitting Heirs."

"Heartfelt, sometimes funny and always engaging, Exit Strategies shares personal reflections and empowering, important life lessons that we all need to know. Each vignette illustrates our resilience and the power of the human spirit and what we are capable of in difficult times."

—Jane Morris, MS, RN. Nursing leader in geriatrics and palliative care

"An excellent resource for families seeking to initiate meaningful conversations about life values and end-of-life choices. I highly recommend this book to anyone looking to engage in these important yet challenging discussions that are deeply significant."

—The Rev. Jon A Overvold, MDiv, BCC Past President, The Association of Professional Chaplains

Exit Strategies

Exit Strategies

LIVING LESSONS *from* DYING PEOPLE

CYNTHIA X. PAN, MD
EXPERT IN HOSPICE AND PALLIATIVE CARE

Copyright © 2024 Cynthia X. Pan

All rights reserved. No part of this publication may be reproduced, distributed, or transmitted in any form or by any means, including photocopying, recording, or other electronic or mechanical methods, without the prior written permission of the publisher, except in the case of brief quotations embodied in critical reviews and certain other noncommercial uses permitted by copyright law. For permission requests, write to the publisher, addressed "Attention: Permissions Coordinator," at the address below.

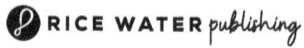

info@cynthiaxpanmd.com

ISBN: 979-8-9910074-0-5 (paperback)
ISBN: 979-8-9910074-1-2 (ebook)
ISBN: 979-8-9910074-2-9 (hardcover)
ISBN: 979-8-9910074-3-6 (audiobook)

Library of Congress Control Number: 2024917020

Ordering Information:
Special discounts are available on quantity purchases by corporations, associations, and others. For details, contact info@cynthiaxpanmd.com

Illustrations by Jiaxi Fu

DEDICATION

To my patients, most of them long gone, but their lessons will live on through me and you!

To my biggest fans: my lovely husband Darrell, my loving mother Hsiang, and my supportive father James.

To my grandma, who gave me my Chinese name, "Happy Heart"

To my two sons, CJ and Christopher, who tell me I am the best mother they ever had! ☺

To those who appreciate Jerry Seinfeld's humorous insight:

> "Surveys show that the number one fear of Americans is public speaking. Number two is death. Death is number two. That means that at a funeral, the average American would rather be in the casket than doing the eulogy."

*** All names are fictitious. Circumstances and stories are taken from my experiences and modified to protect the privacy of the patients.

Table of Contents

Introduction 1
Chapter 1: It's Not Cocktail Party Conversation,
　　　　　 but It Should Be 15
Chapter 2: Advance Directives. 27
Chapter 3: Food. 45
Chapter 4: Music at the End of Life 69
Chapter 5: Family Meetings. 77
Chapter 6: Total Pain and the Vortex. 95
Chapter 7: Hospice 113
Chapter 8: Terri Schiavo—A Missed Opportunity
　　　　　 for Advance Directives 121
Chapter 9: Religion and Spirituality 127
Chapter 10: Birthdays 149
Chapter 11: Using the Right Words 159
Chapter 12: Palliative Extubation: Disconnecting
　　　　　　from the Ventilator. 163
Chapter 13: Facing My Mortality During My
　　　　　　COVID Illness 181
Chapter 14: Find an Excuse to Celebrate or
　　　　　　Make a Bucket List 193

Chapter 15: People Who Plan Their Own
　　　　　　　Funerals 203
Chapter 16: Capacity 215
Chapter 17: Sex in the City ... at the End of Life .227
Chapter 18: You Are My Final Doctor 239
Chapter 19: Discussing Advance Directives with
　　　　　　　My Parents and Brother 253
Chapter 20: The EOL Passport for Our Last
　　　　　　　Journey. 269
Appendix: Additional Resources 281
Acknowledgments 289
Notes 301

Introduction

WE HAVE A PROBLEM IN THIS COUNTRY.

Terminally ill persons have important things to say to their families but don't share them because they're afraid and lack the language to express these strong emotions. Important things like their end-of-life wishes, personal preferences about how to spend their remaining days, and messages they want to send and say to their loved ones often go unspoken. The fear is real. Too many people fear expressing their thoughts and feelings lest their families and friends judge them, or think less of them, or break out crying uncontrollably. Sometimes dying people feel ashamed of their illness or decline, or their families and communities feel ashamed to let outsiders know about a family member's illness.

Terminally ill persons may want to express their feelings but not know how. Their families may not be willing to listen and instead want to (falsely) reassure them that all is well. This is not a new phenomenon. Leo

Tolstoy, the famed Russian novelist, wrote about this in 1886 in his novella entitled *The Death of Ivan Ilyich*. However, during these complex and challenging times, there are important opportunities for growth, meaning, and liberation if we can open ourselves up to them.

The solution is to normalize and openly discuss end-of-life issues so that terminally ill persons and their families can use their limited time left together to communicate what's most important to them, and so families will not live with regrets after the terminally ill person has died. Just think about what happened on 9/11. When the passengers on the plane realized that the plane was heading for the World Trade Center towers and destruction and that they would die, many of them pulled out their cell phones and called their loved ones to say goodbye and tell them "I love you" one last time.

THE IMPORTANCE OF PERSONAL WISHES

What may be important to one person may differ from what is important to another. Only by communicating

Introduction

about personal wishes can we know what they are. Even husbands and wives who have been married for many years may not know what their spouse's wishes and preferences are. I know because I experienced this when I was severely ill with COVID-19. More about that later.

FROM FEAR TO HEALING

In my experience as a hospice and palliative care physician speaking with thousands of terminally ill patients, the important things boil down to three buckets:

1. Maintaining function and independence.
2. Optimizing quality of life even when quantity is limited.
3. Maximizing time left with loved ones.

In life, too often we are afraid to speak up and ask for what we want. Receiving a terminal diagnosis, while devastating, is also a golden opportunity to speak our mind and ask for what we want and need so we can freely individualize and personalize our own end-of-life care. Now is the time to learn a new language: a language of love, candor, humor, and advocacy. No need to wait!

I know the solution works because I have cared for thousands of terminally ill patients and witnessed their transformation from fear and anxiety to being able to openly discuss their feelings, build more meaningful relationships with their families, and promote spiritual and emotional healing at the end of life. Of course, I have also met others who never took that step, and those are the ones who suffered the most.

TOMORROW COULD BE HERE SOONER THAN YOU THINK

I often work with patients to help them understand their outlook—and all of the care options available to them—so they can make choices that best align with their wishes. One such patient I was asked to visit (to provide a palliative care consult) had end-stage liver cancer. He ended up in the hospital because he had a

Introduction

lot of ascites, or fluid in his abdomen. Everybody had a sense that he was pretty sick. But when we talked to the patient, he suggested he was okay.

"When I get out of here, I'm gonna get additional treatment. It's not that bad. I'm walking around. I'm gonna go see my oncologist," he said.

My fellow and I weren't so sure—but we didn't want to discourage or mislead him.

"All right. Not for now, but for the future, can we talk a little bit about hospice care? Just so you know about it," I said.

He agreed, so we talked about hospice. Afterward, I called his oncologist to learn more information—I wanted to make sure everyone was on the same page. As it turned out, the patient had received lots of treatment, but his body wasn't responding to it. The doctors had done everything they could to stop his cancer from spreading. But at this point, his disease had progressed.

"He should be in hospice," the oncologist told me (a lot of times you don't get such a frank assessment).

Exit Strategies

When we revisited the patient, the medical team alerted us that his kidney function had worsened. He was frustrated—he wanted to be discharged from the hospital and go home. His wife was there to visit him, and I introduced myself.

"We don't want palliative care," his wife said. "We want to go home and to get more treatment."

"That's understandable," I told her. "I just had a discussion with the oncologist. Can I tell you what's going on?"

"Sure."

"Should we talk about this here with your husband or outside?"

"Let's talk outside, because he gets confused." Confusion and disorientation are common side effects for people with liver cancer. After we stepped outside, I told her what the oncologist said, and she was taken aback.

"I can see how frustrating this situation is for you because he wants to go home, and now he can't. It's difficult to stabilize things that won't stabilize. But

Introduction

by the time the kidneys get affected from the liver, it's end stage."

She focused on that term: *end stage*. She called her daughter on the phone and told her the news, too, and the daughter asked me questions that I dutifully answered. The patient's wife and daughter accused the doctors of lying to them—but in reality, people tried to tell them about the situation all along. They just didn't want to hear it.

As difficult as it all was, I needed them to hear my message.

"He could stay another twelve days in the hospital and not leave, because none of his markers are going to normalize," I warned them. "If you don't want to recognize that, he's probably going to be stuck here."

"We've always said that if he's terminal, then he wants to go home," his wife told me. "And that's what I want."

"This is the window," I told her. "Because if he gets sicker, he may really not be able to go home. And if he goes home, he'll still be able to visit his oncologist."

"Okay."

"Okay. Let's make sure we are on the same page: accepting the fact that he's terminally ill, and even though his lab numbers are not normal, you want him to go home. That's a more important goal than his labs. Is that what we're saying?"

"Yes."

"All right. We'll tell the medical team and I'll call his attending physician. We'll plan to release him tomorrow."

We started to talk about hospice, and they were not interested. "We want him home. We don't want him to be in hospice," they said.

"Well, did you know that hospice is mostly at home? That's what we're talking about. If his goal is to be at home and stay home and not come back multiple times, then at-home hospice is the best option," I said.

They were surprised—and hopeful—to learn about the opportunities available to him with at-home hospice. I gave the patient's family members

Introduction

information about nearby hospices, offered advice for talking to his oncologist, and there we were.

People who don't want to think about the end of their life often say they'll worry about things in the future when they come, *someday*. But that day could come sooner than you think. The future could be here faster than you know it.

Keep an open mind. It takes courage. I know you can do it.

And if you can't or don't want to, that's okay, too.

After all, this is a free country.

EMBRACING THE SADNESS AND HUMOR

I am a medical expert who cares for and advises patients facing the end of their lives. I mediate meaningful and sensitive conversations with their families. I was not born with these skills! I struggled with my own insecurities, fears, uncertainties, and imposter syndrome. Through my training and introspective practice, I learned the language of acknowledging emotions, validating my own and other people's concerns, and the importance of real listening. I learned when to set boundaries and when to let go. I now teach other medical professionals how to practice active listening and how to speak concisely and not overwhelm patients and their families.

Practicing palliative care (which deals with serious illness, relieving symptoms and suffering, when the main cause of the condition is often irreversible) reminds me that life is short, and I really cannot take myself too seriously. The best way to get through tough times may be to approach it with a sense of humor. We do not give our fellow human beings enough credit. I am always amazed at the sense of humor that people display, even when they are terminally ill. On the other hand, people may use humor as a coping mechanism to deflect the fear or create a distraction from needed conversations.

For example, Ben was a retired cook with progressive cancer and self-reported low literacy. When the doctors relayed information, they mainly spoke with his son instead of him. When I spoke with Ben and his

Introduction

wife, Ben told me he wanted the doctors to tell <u>him</u> about his medical condition and his treatment plan. He said with a laugh, "I want everyone to be honest with me. If it's goodbye, then it's goodbye." He brought a smile to all of us. When people are faced with challenges, they rise to the task. You can form very intense relationships in a short time. Many profound and intense exchanges happen during initial introductions without having gone far in our conversations.

WHAT I HOPE YOU LEARN FROM READING THIS BOOK

This is a book about how end of life can be filled with meaning, growth, humor, and people helping people. I want this book to be positive and show you that end of life still has "LIFE" in it! I meet so many people who can teach and give so much, even as they are dying. It's weird sometimes driving around in Queens. I pass by houses where someone was alive a few months ago, and now they've died. I sometimes wonder if we live among spirits all the time but just do not know it. It's pretty humbling.

Exit Strategies

I wrote this for terminally ill people and their families and loved ones who wish to appreciate how much every day matters in the new light that facing mortality creates. It is for people who are willing to face their fears and anxieties and find liberation and joy on the other side of the terminal illness tunnel. It is for people who, despite the setbacks and challenges of terminal illness, want to continue learning and growing, have a laugh each day, and let go a little. You will notice that I am using the words "die" or "dying" instead of sugarcoating it with "passed away."

In this book, I present stories of patients and their families who struggle with everyday concerns and come to appreciate life's little things—all while facing mortality. Each story features an everyday topic but with an end-of-life twist. These topics include sex, eating, music, birthdays, celebrations, pain, suffering, journeys, and more. I share several stories about advance care planning, which means sharing end-of-life wishes and preferences with loved ones, to ensure that you receive care that aligns with your personal values, goals, and preferences. Often, advance care planning is a very important but missed opportunity. As a matter of fact, the national

Introduction

motto for advance care planning is, *"It often seems too early, until it's too late."* Each chapter concludes with lessons—important topics and pearls that I hope you will keep in mind and talk to someone about.

I wrote *Exit Strategies* to reassure you that *you are not alone*. I want to help people have peace of mind as they—or their loved ones—face the prospect of end-of-life care. I also want to normalize discussing end-of-life matters. So many times I have seen both my patients struggle from not knowing how to talk about their end-of-life wishes and preferences with their families while they were still able to, and their families suffer when they desperately wanted to know the patients' wishes when it's suddenly too late. Many terminally ill persons do not know about their options and resources, so they suffer unnecessarily. The end-of-life experience does not have to be that way. I want to help you turn missed opportunities into golden opportunities for meaningful conversations, expressing and acknowledging emotions, and validating yourselves and your loved ones. I feel that together, as a team, we can break the mold and liberate ourselves to both speak our minds and actively listen.

I hope that you will use the stories in this book as icebreakers to start conversations with yourself and your loved ones about what you want and don't want at the end of your life. I hope you will learn from our predecessors and transform the dying process into a living legacy process.

And remember: End of life is still part of life! Even at the end of life, you can still find meaning, humor, and the strength to help others!

CHAPTER 1

It's Not Cocktail Party Conversation, but It Should Be

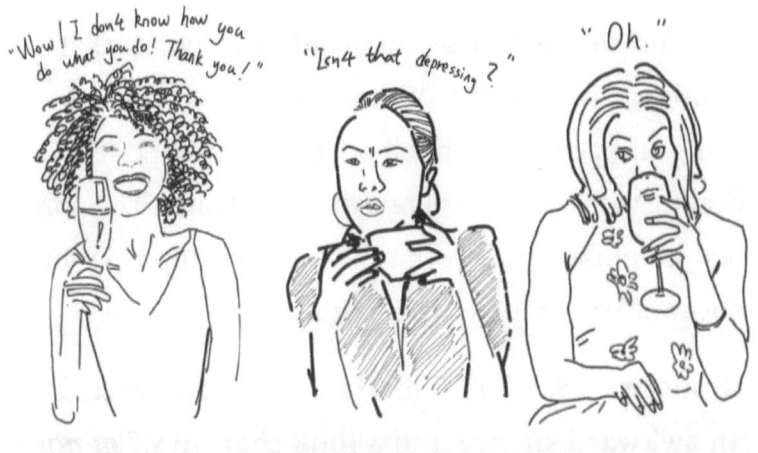

WHENEVER I TELL PEOPLE THAT I'M A HOSPICE and palliative care doctor, I usually get one of three reactions.

Response #1: *"Isn't that depressing?"*

I want to firmly say, "It's not!" Sad sometimes, yes. Depressing to me, no. Hospice and palliative care can be very rewarding and meaningful because I get to help people when they need it most. I also possess the temperament and training to do it, so why not?

Response #2: *"Wow. I don't know how you do what you do. Thank you!"*

I am so touched by this kind of response that I thank them profusely. We can keep a conversation going and people often tell me their own experiences dealing with seriously ill or dying loved ones. The normal response to the work I do is sincere appreciation once you've experienced it firsthand.

Response #3: *"Oh."* **This is usually followed by an awkward silence and a look that says,** *I'm not sure what.*

When this occurs, one of us makes an excuse and walks away. Awkward!

I've gotten so much flak for practicing hospice and end-of-life care. Colleagues have called me "the

It's Not Cocktail Party Conversation, but It Should Be

Grim Reaper" or "Angel of Death," which really stings. *What the hell? I'm a doctor just like you!*

End of life is still part of life, and we shouldn't abandon people at this stage. At some point, we're all going to be there ourselves. When I began facing mean comments and awkward responses, at first I tried to defend myself. "This is what I do," I'd tell others. But in truth, I didn't want to have to defend myself. So after a while, I decided I wasn't going to say anything. Maybe I just wouldn't talk about my work even though it's very important to me. People are interested in orthopedics, emergency medicine, or cardiology—those are things people can understand. But when you say, "palliative care" or "hospice," there's often a different reaction.

Keeping quiet wasn't the right answer, either. It took me a long time to come up with a comeback to the "Angel of Death" comments—something thoughtful and insightful.

So today when somebody calls me "Angel of Death," I say, "You have the wrong 'D.' It's 'Angel of Dignity.' Our patients are typically going to die, and my role is protecting their dignity and upholding their wishes. So if I know what their wishes are and I can help contribute to their dignity, that's what I'm going to do."

I've also found a new way to break the ice. I smile and teasingly say, "Are you scared yet?"

MY JOURNEY

I didn't set out to be a palliative care doctor. But reflecting on my life, I feel blessed that my parents chose (or "voluntold" me) medicine as my profession.

I come from a fairly traditional Chinese family. In my reserved upbringing, things were often "unsaid" rather than said, but I always knew I was surrounded by love. My mother was always there to support and help me with my homework—especially when I was up late at night to finish an assignment. On the other hand, there were things that were glossed over and not discussed. One example of this is what to expect for my first menstrual period. When it happened, I was in shock and paralyzed with fear. I hid it and dealt

It's Not Cocktail Party Conversation, but It Should Be

with it for several days before gathering the courage to speak with her.

"Mom, I think I'm dying," I told her.

When I explained what happened, she burst out laughing. Feeling completely indignant and shocked, I questioned why she was laughing at the horrifying news. Yes, that's how I learned about menstruations.

During my high school years in Brooklyn, New York, I wasn't permitted to drink alcohol or hang out late with my friends. If I talked with my male classmates on the phone, my father would train my younger brother to eavesdrop, and interrupt the call to say that the conversation is over if we weren't talking about homework.

My high school years were so sheltered that when I attended college at Harvard, I had no idea what the party scenes were like. During my freshman week at college, the guys living downstairs from my suite came up to ask for donations for a "cake party." I gladly donated $5 and was quite impressed by how civilized Harvard University was. *Guys organizing cake parties?* When the night of the cake party came,

I was aghast to see more drunken young people lining the floors than I could ever imagine. When I timidly asked where the cake was, someone pointed me in the direction of the beer keg. That's when I learned the difference between "cake" parties and "keg" parties!

Medicine helped me expand my narrow definition of "normal," too. As a third-year medical student, I interviewed a male patient who was a veteran. I dutifully asked a full history, including his alcohol intake. He told me that he drank "a little," but emphatically denied he was an alcoholic. He stated that sometimes he needed to take a drink in the morning and had a bottle under his bed. For him, that was "normal."

When I presented the case to my attending physician I reiterated these facts, emphasizing that the patient was not an alcoholic, as he stated. My attending physician laughed so hard he almost fell off his chair. That's when I learned what an "eye-opener" was in terms of diagnosing alcoholism.

Then I met my husband and his loud, party-loving, and very caring family. With a mix of Italian, Polish, and German heritages commingled with American expressionism, I didn't know what hit me. I would hide in the corner of the house terrified, unsure if what people told me was a joke or a serious statement.

With some time and after getting to know my husband's family, I learned to be less serious about myself and the world and how to loosen up. I learned to use jokes and humor as a way to manage social anxiety. I learned to accept the spectrum of normal interactions, which included cursing, laughing hard, freaking out, sarcasm, screaming, or stone silence.

MY SHIFT TO PALLIATIVE CARE

As I approached my career, I really didn't know what my medical specialty would be. I knew I wanted to go into internal medicine, which involved working with lots of older people. I also had an interest in pain management, which turned out to be a major part of palliative care.

Working with older patients made me think about my grandmother, who I was very close with growing up. She's the one who gave me my name, Xin Xin, which means "happy heart" in Chinese characters. When I was little, I lived next door to my grandmother. Almost daily, and certainly every weekend, I would visit grandma and sit with her, listening to her stories about fleeing China, raising five children, and becoming a government leader. I didn't realize how meaningful it was at the time but looking back now—wow!

I also have fond memories of my grandmother hosting parties and hiring a catering chef who made the most delicious butterfly shrimp. I would organize my brother and cousins to go to the kitchen and sneak some of the butterfly shrimp until the chef got nervous about running out of food and chased us all out of the kitchen. Grandmother would also make us delicious Shanghai-style noodles, and my cousins and I would have a contest to see who could put the most hot spice sauce in the noodles. Though it was cause us to sweat like crazy, it was so much fun.

My grandmother lived in Taiwan and got sick when I was in medical school. When she was dying, I couldn't really visit her, and because of this, there was a lack of closure. Even all these years later, I can still close my eyes and see the image of her standing by the gate at the airport waving goodbye to me. It was one of the last times I saw her.

In some ways, working with hospice patience makes me feel like maybe I could be there for other patients in a way I couldn't help my grandmother.

I plunged into palliative care after completing my residency and geriatrics fellowship (specializing in the care of older people). Becoming a palliative care doctor thrust me into a world of patients facing serious illness, family dramas, unraveling relationships, tensions, angry outbursts, lack of communication, and family members walking out of meetings. On the other hand, there was brutal honesty, refreshing resilience, tender loving, and amazing courage. I embraced all these emotions as my definition of "normal" continued to expand.

Palliative care can be an "unspeakable" topic because terminal illness is scary. Everything seems so final and grim. The sadness and thought of losing a dear loved one are overwhelming! Then again, I was once told that "If you feel pain, it means you're alive."

What a way to reframe! Hospice and palliative care are not your usual cocktail conversation topics, but maybe they should be.

DEFINING PALLIATIVE CARE

Palliative care can be defined as providing team-based care for people (and their families) who have serious illnesses. Serious illness usually brings stress for the patient as well as the family and sometimes even the community. You can think of palliative care as an extra layer of support in a time of great stress. Palliative care teams usually try to find out and support each patient's wishes and preferences according to their values, understand what matters most to them, and facilitate a meaningful discussion between the patient and the family.

Palliative care is the umbrella term. Under it comes hospice, which is a benefit and program for patients who have a life expectancy of six months or less. Hospice care provides care for patients at the end of life and is covered by Medicare and many other insurances. It provides home visits to help keep patients comfortable and supported while guiding families and caregivers. Home visits are done by a team of hospice doctors, nurses, nurse practitioners, social workers, chaplains, volunteers, and hospice aides. Unlike regular home care, which answers phones from 9 a.m. to 5 p.m., hospices answer phone calls 24/7 and through the weekends. Staff members also make emergency visits to patients who have active symptoms. Having been trained in a variety of hospital settings, I was shocked to learn how much can be done in a home hospice setting to keep our patients comfortable.

LESSONS

- Your help is needed to make palliative care and end of life easier to discuss.
- Palliative care is team-based care for people who have serious illnesses. Palliative care is an umbrella term and includes hospice care.
- If I run into you at a cocktail party, be nice to me. Please don't call me the "Angel of Death." It's Angel of Dignity—thank you very much!

CHAPTER 2

Advance Directives

I'VE DISCUSSED ADVANCE DIRECTIVES—OR A patient's wishes about their care options in case they can't make decisions for themselves at some point in the future—for many years. Sometimes, those conversations don't go as planned and can be quite difficult for all involved.

Patients facing end-of-life care need to be courageous enough to think about it in advance and ask their doctors to talk about advance directives. Ultimately, the type of end-of-life care they receive is up to them. They can either accept or reject treatment, or decide the specific treatment options that matter most to them.

FORMING A RELATIONSHIP

When I have conversations with patients about their advance directives and wishes, it's really about forming a relationship. You can't just walk into a room and say, "Well, you don't have much time left, what do you want?" Forming that bond is especially important where I work in Queens, New York. Patients come from hundreds of different countries, and many require an interpreter to communicate. Many of these patients don't trust doctors to begin with—especially if they're not from the patient's background.

My job is to make sure I ask patients questions and learn more about them, which helps to develop as strong of a bond as possible. Some of these questions include:

- Where were you born or raised?
- What type of work do (or did) you do?
- Who are your closest to?
- What is your family support like?
- Are you spiritual or religious?
- What are the things that matter most to you?
- What brings you joy and meaning?

Lots of doctors use big medical words that most people don't understand. When that happens, patients are prone to get lost and will shy away from asking you any questions, as they don't want to feel stupid for asking about the wrong thing.

My heart goes out to people facing end-of-life care. It's possible that some of these patients feel like giving up, that whatever they do doesn't matter, and that it will all be over soon anyway. They might also be embarrassed or in denial.

However, the way I see it is this is their chance to speak up and make sure their feelings are heard! This is the time to lay out a game plan for their remaining days—to make the most of the time they have. For me, it's an important time of life that shouldn't be overlooked.

MR. M

A few years ago, I met with Mr. M, an elderly gentleman with lung disease. He was suffering from emphysema, lung scarring (or fibrosis), and now pneumonia.

He was on BIPAP, a machine with a tight mask that pushes air and oxygen into his lungs. With BIPAP, it's hard to talk and eat because of the tight mask that needs to be worn. When I spoke to him, he was barely able to get his words out. My fellow (specialist doctor in training) and I were asked to explain his advance directives to him and were told that he was all alone. Apparently, his daughter was his healthcare proxy, but no one could find her, and Mr. M was residing in a nursing home.

We went to his hospital room, greeted him, and introduced ourselves. We asked how he was doing. "Okay," Mr. M said.

Since we wanted to get to know him a little better, we sat down on the chairs next to his hospital bed and asked him if he understood his medical conditions and how he came to be admitted to the hospital. Mr. M told us that he knew he had emphysema, as he was a longtime smoker. He knew that now that he was in a nursing home he had to stop smoking. He said he didn't really miss it. He went to the nursing home after his wife died because he couldn't take care of himself anymore. At the nursing

Advance Directives

home, his meals were taken care of, staff would help transport him to different areas, there were social activities and games, and he even made a couple of acquaintances. When we asked if it was okay to talk about advance directives with him and if he knew what that meant, he said, "Yes. It's when they decide if you're going to live or die."

"Wow," I said. "That's very direct. I guess we can start there."

"I don't mince words. Direct is good," he replied.

I took a deep breath and began. "Mr. M, your lungs are not functioning well. You have three hits on your lungs, and two of them are not reversible. Do you know what I'm saying?"

"Yes, I understand," he replied.

"This BIPAP machine that you're on, it's the last straw. If this one doesn't work, you may have to go on life support machines and have a tube inserted down your throat to breathe artificially for you," I explained.

"I don't want that. No artificial machines," he said firmly.

"Not even as a trial? See how you do?" I asked.

"No. They asked me that at the nursing home. I've seen people like that. What's the point?" He sighed.

"Let's step back a bit. Could you tell me, what are some things that bring your life joy, that are meaningful to you?"

"It's the little things at this point. The basics. If it's a sunny day out and someone can wheel me outside for fresh air, that makes my day. I used to love going hiking. I guess my hiking days are over," he said wistfully.

"Thank you for sharing that, Mr. M," I said sincerely. "I can't imagine what it must be like to be such an active man and to now be cooped up inside a nursing home."

"Nothing I can do about it," he shrugged.

"What about family? Do you have family around here?" I asked.

"I had a daughter but she died. She lived in Pennsylvania. At first they were afraid to tell me—the nursing home people. But eventually I found out. I mean, how long can you hide something like that?" He sneered.

Advance Directives

"I'm so sorry to hear that. It's horrible to lose your daughter." Now I understood why no one could reach her.

"Yes, thank you. So now I have no one. I mean, I have a son-in-law—she was married," he added.

Curious, I asked, "Are you in touch with your son-in-law?"

"No. I didn't like him to begin with. Now that she's dead, we're not in touch." He said this in a very matter of fact way.

"So, Mr. M, since your daughter is no longer with us, it's more important than ever that we talk about your advance directives while your mind is strong and clear. We want to make sure our medical treatments are in line with what you want and what's important to you. And only *you* can tell us what you want. Our job is to support you."

"Okay, I'm all ears." He smiled.

"You already told us that you don't want to be on an artificial life support machine for breathing. What about if your heart stops? Would you want to go peacefully or have doctors and nurses come and thump on your chest, give you CPR, and electrical shocks to try to revive you?" I stumbled around these questions awkwardly.

"No, it's okay. I'll pass on that."

"That means, in medical terms, you prefer to be DNR and DNI—do not resuscitate and do not intubate. That tells me you want to die naturally. Is that accurate?" I confirmed.

"That's right. What else?"

"Well, what if your condition gets worse and you get weaker, and you can't eat naturally or normally, would you want your doctor to give you a feeding tube? This would be put surgically into your stomach."

"I'm not sure. Let's talk about that when we get there," he replied.

"Unfortunately, by then it will be too late," I said. "Most people at that stage will not be able to think clearly or even speak or communicate." At this time I was getting nervous for him.

"I don't see the big deal. Why don't we do this. If I can talk, then ask me. If I cannot talk, then *don't do it*," he replied.

I thought about what he said. Wow! Could it be so simple? So binary?

If I can talk, then ask me.

If I cannot talk, then *don't do it*.

Right now, at least in New York state, the default path is this: If I can talk, ask me. If I cannot talk, then *do it*.

The default path is to assume everyone wants to live in whatever condition in order to extend their lives—even if it causes you to end up in a vegetative state.

But what if we could change the default mode? Instead, we should ask our patients: What is your default mode? If you can talk, then we will definitely ask you. If you cannot talk because you are terminally ill, then should we *do it*, or *don't do it?* Encouraging this conversation between our patients and their families is what's best for everyone.

But let's get back to Mr. M.

"Wow, you're brilliant. And yes, I agree with you. If you can talk, then we will definitely ask you. If you cannot talk because you are terminally ill, then we *won't do it*. We'll let you pass naturally, peacefully. Correct?" I asked to confirm.

"You got it, doc!" he agreed.

"Would you be willing to put this down in writing? NYS has a MOLST form to document these discussions. We will give you a copy."

"Of course. Thanks doc!"

WHEN FAMILY MEMBERS DON'T HEED A PATIENT'S ADVANCE DIRECTIVES

Relatives are often left to make decisions for a patient who isn't able to choose on their own. But sometimes even when a patient is able to make decisions, a family member can hijack or overpower their loved one's wishes.

Advance Directives

We treated an Italian gentleman with advanced lung disease who wanted to be DNR (do not resuscitate) and DNI (do not intubate). He didn't want to be on machines and simply wanted to be on home hospice.

Unfortunately, his wife would reverse these decisions.

"Don't listen to him. He's talking crazy. I know he can be treated," she said. "He needs to be full code. You need to do everything you can. And if he gets on the machine, you need to keep him alive for as long as possible so he can come back. And I don't want to hear any talk of hospice."

Any time we spoke about his wishes, she would get upset and start throwing people out of the room.

I visited them with my fellow to get his basic history and condition. During this time, the wife was very nice and forthcoming. That is, until we got to the sensitive topic of treatment options.

The line of conversation wasn't unrealistic. The patient was really, really sick. We always have to ask if somebody wants to be intubated on the machines because this could happen—in this case, the patient was in the ICU and his breathing wasn't good. We wanted to know what we should do, and what *he would want*, if his condition worsened.

"I don't want to be intubated," the patient said.

"No, he has to be intubated," the wife immediately responded.

The patient closed his eyes and tried to calm his nerves, or perhaps ease his frustrations.

"You know what, I don't want to talk about this anymore. This is very depressing. And don't you see that you're making me upset? Why are you asking me these questions?" the wife asked.

The patient opened his eyes.

"I have a question," he said. "What about home hospice? I want to know more about that."

I was encouraged by his question.

"That type of care is for people who have end-stage disease," I told him.

"Yes, I want home hospice," he told me. "I'm a grown man, but I can't do anything for myself. I need somebody to turn me. I poop in bed, I pee in bed, I'm a burden to my family." His statement was so profound.

The room became silent, and his wife became tearful.

"Wow, that's a lot," I told him. "I give you a lot of credit for talking about this so openly in front of your family. This is important."

Before we had a chance to explore his wishes further, his wife responded.

"No, this is no good. Stop asking him all these questions. You're upsetting me. There's no home hospice. I'm not gonna take him home on home hospice, and he's going to be intubated. And you ladies need to leave right now," she said.

"You know, I feel really bad because I know the patient is thinking about something that's different from the way you feel," I said, at which point the patient's family—but not the patient—asked us to leave.

I asked the patient what he wished to do.

He closed his eyes again before responding.

"I guess I'll go with my wife's plan," he said.

"Do you want us to come back at some point?"

"No, don't come back," she said.

"Okay, we're going to leave. But if you change your mind in the future and want us to come back, we can always come back. And we don't want to upset anyone. But I just want to say that you should really listen to the patient," I said.

Cases like this are difficult—the patient is saying one thing, the family is saying another. We cannot speak up for people who don't speak up for themselves. All we can do is witness and document the situation. It's a lot of moral distress for us as doctors and health care professionals!

Typically, the patient doesn't have capacity and their relatives are speaking on their behalf. It's not often that the patient can make decisions about their care and they're being overruled by their family members.

I want to help patients, but I don't want to be in between a husband and wife and their very different perspectives about advance directives.

ADVANCE DIRECTIVES AND DIFFERENT CULTURES

Having an end-of-life plan in advance is a Western, Anglo-Saxon concept. There are cultural reasons why people from other backgrounds don't always rely on or embrace advance directives.

For example, where Western cultures are more future-oriented, many Asian cultures tend to be more past-oriented and focused on history.[1] It's about honoring your ancestry and respecting the elderly because they represent your past. In that context, the topic of advance directives may be viewed by some as disrespectful to your relatives—but we try to reframe that viewpoint because advance directives are really about respecting their wishes and helping them achieve their care goals.

Similarly, many Latino cultures are more present-focused. They want to know what is happening today and now. Whatever happened yesterday is gone. Whatever may happen tomorrow is not here yet. You

---

[1] Jack K.H. Pun, "Communication About Advance Directives and Advance Care Planning in an East Asian Cultural Context: A Systematic Review," *Oncology Nursing Forum* 49, no. 1 (2022): 58–70, https://doi.org/10.1188/22.ONF.58-70.

may have heard the concept of "mañana," which can mean tomorrow or an unspecified time in the future. It is common for Latino patients to put off until mañana something they do not want to face today, such as advance directives.

While cultural influences could impact a patient's desire to discuss advance directives, each patient should know that the option is available for them. Cultural time-orientation is only one element of a person's identity, and each patient is an individual with their own care choices and options to choose from.

LESSONS

- Advance directives are a chance for your wishes to be heard! Think of it as a game plan or an insurance policy for the end of your life.
- Don't be afraid to ask your doctor to spend a little time getting to know you as a person! Feel free to tell your doctor something unique or personal about you, to form a more trusting relationship.

Advance Directives

- Don't be afraid to start the conversation about advance directives with your doctor. You can write a letter to your doctor using the Stanford Letter Project template (https://med.stanford.edu/letter/about.html).
- What is your default mode?
- If you can talk, then we will definitely ask you.
- If you cannot talk because you are terminally ill, then should we do it, or don't do it?

CHAPTER 3

Food

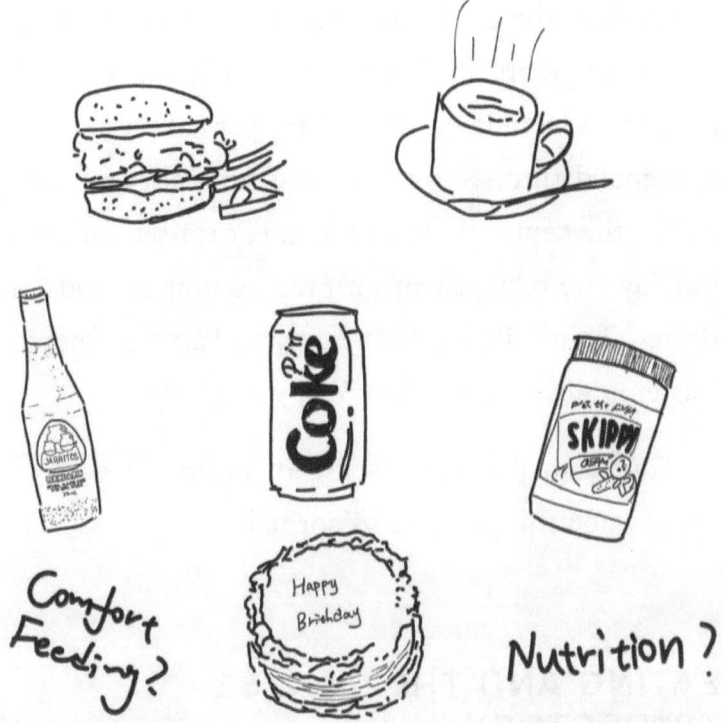

FOOD IS A BASIC NECESSITY. SOME OF US "EAT to live," while others "live to eat." You can decide which appeals more to you!

Food is also highly symbolic and represents love and caring. Whether we gather for celebrations or mourning, food is usually involved. My brother still remembers the delicious lamb chops from my wedding many years ago! Many would not think of celebrating a birthday without a proper cake. One year, I attended three Shivas and two funerals, and food was at the center in all of them. For various cultural holidays, we relate them with representative foods or dishes. Think Thanksgiving turkey, Passover matzo, Easter lamb, or Lunar New Year dumplings.

Food can provide a sense of normalcy, even at times when things aren't so normal.

EATING AND THE ILLNESS TRAJECTORY

A common path for patients facing the end of a terminal illness is loss of appetite (anorexia) and unintentional weight loss (cachexia). Anorexia and cachexia are expected symptoms in the illness trajectory. But most people don't think about that or know about it.

When a loved one who used to enjoy eating and sampling various cuisines loses their appetite and starts losing weight, it raises huge alarms for the family members. Often, we don't realize that the goals we set for healthy people are not realistic for those who have end-stage diseases.

There are many factors to consider involving food and a patient's condition—but for those facing hospice and end-of-life care, outside-the-box thinking is important. It's given me so much joy to see my patients happy over a simple bite or sip of their favorite food or drink, without having to argue with well-intentioned people around them.

CHICKEN SANDWICH

"You want a bite?" asked David, my patient. He was lying in bed, his bedsheets sprinkled with skin debris. He was ill with cancer and could not manage his daily care, much less clean his linens. Luckily, he was able to call out and order food. On the day I visited, he had just received a delivery of a massive chicken cutlet sandwich. He was noshing on half and offered me the other half.

"No, thank you," I replied.

"C'mon, try some! It's really good," David insisted.

"Thank you, but I just had a *big* lunch," I declined, trying to be polite. "May I sit down?"

"Yeah, of course. Pull up a chair."

Opening my laptop, I began to ask him questions about his pain—symptoms like breathing, appetite, constipation, anxiety, sadness, and other factors. David answered my questions, but clearly his focus was on his chicken sandwich. I could see how much joy he got from savoring the sandwich, and it made me happy to watch him.

Even in the face of a difficult prognosis, he was making the most of every bite.

Food

PEANUT BUTTER

Alan was homebound and lived in a small studio apartment that he couldn't clean or take care of. Looking around the place, I wasn't sure where I could lay down my house-calls bag. Alan said he was hungry and asked if I could get him some peanut butter from his pantry.

"Of course! Where is your pantry?" I asked.

He pointed to the narrow hallway leading to the kitchen. Alan was set up in a dimly lit living room and was laying in his hospital bed. Inside the dark-paneled pantry was a brand-new jar of peanut butter. I could see the oil layer freely floating.

"Please bring me a spoon! You can get yourself a spoon too," Alan shouted from the living room.

Back in the living room, I found a stool where I placed my medical bag. I handed him the jar and a spoon as a cockroach leisurely crept across the far wall. Alan thoroughly enjoyed his peanut butter, licking the spoon's hollow and back side. He looked comfortable and shared that the hospice nurse who visited the day before had increased his pain medication, and with his pain better controlled, his appetite returned.

He also told me his sister had called to check in on him, and he was happy to hear from her. He was worried about lack of groceries, as he could not go out anymore. Luckily, his neighbor stopped by with his favorite kind of peanut butter.

I suggested that it might be a good time to allow a hospice aide to come in and help him. This would include shopping for simple groceries, helping him keep clean, and straightening the apartment a bit.

"I know, I know. I've been thinking about it. I think I will give it a try," he said.

"Do you want to talk to your nurse or social worker about it? Or should I just ask the office to find an aide for you?" I asked.

"I trust you. Just send someone. But please send me someone good and responsible," he emphasized. "Are you sure you don't want some peanut butter? It's the best brand out there!"

I found a clean plastic spoon and scooped up some peanut butter. It was delicious!

END-OF-LIFE NUTRITION STANDARDS

In this country, we have healthy people nutrition guidelines, but we fall behind in setting reasonable nutrition guidelines and expectations at end of life. Healthy eating guidelines that are recommended for the general population are not appropriate when you're tired, lying in bed, not working, not running around, not hungry, and already eating less than usual. For people at the end of life, we need to reframe and reset our expectations. The benefits of eating and drinking should always outweigh the risks and burdens to a person who is unwell. Reframing should occur around the types of foods, consistency of foods and drinks, amount expected to be eaten, and a loosening of food restrictions. Many hospice care agencies have certified dietitian nutritionists who can advise and counsel patients about nutrition and foods at this stage of life.

AVERSIVE FEEDING BEHAVIORS

I've seen so many patients sent in for care from homes or nursing homes because they stopped eating or because they were not eating as well and were losing weight. Sometimes these were temporary or reversible symptoms of an acute illness. But many times, we find ourselves seeing a patient with advanced stages of dementia or some other condition who has been losing weight and not eating well for quite some time.

They become visibly thinner or appear wasted, state they have no appetite, or refuse to eat when offered meals. They might have become weaker or have fallen down. In patients with advanced dementia, there are symptoms that comprise the syndrome of "aversive feeding behaviors." These include resisting or being indifferent to food, clenching the mouth and not allowing to be fed, not being able to manage the food bolus properly once it is in the mouth (oral phase dysphagia), or aspirating when swallowing (pharyngeal phase dysphagia).

Such behavioral troubles are perceived as a heavy burden by family caregivers who may be stressed, depressed, and socially isolated from caregiving responsibilities. For patients with dementia, caregivers may spend extraordinary amounts of time just trying to feed their loved ones. An excellent book that I highly recommend is *The 36-Hour Day: A Family Guide to Caring for People Who Have Alzheimer Disease and Other Dementias*, written by Nancy L. Mace, MA, and Peter V. Rabins, MD, MPH.

I've heard countless family members say, "Please make him/her eat. If only he/she would eat more, then they will get better." The problem is, trouble eating is an expected part of the illness and will seldom get better. Think about when you get a bad case of the flu or COVID—do you have a good appetite? The difference is, at end of life, the appetite and weight loss are there to stay!

When someone has advanced illness and trouble swallowing or eating, doctors will ask speech and swallow therapists to evaluate the patient. To be safe, the therapists may recommend NPO (Latin for "nil per os," which translates into "nothing by mouth") or some alternative way of feeding—like a surgically inserted feeding tube (PEG). For patients who have advanced dementia and have already lost the ability to speak, walk, or complete routine self-care activities (like bathing or personal hygiene), a PEG will not reverse these consequences. Consequences of advanced dementia may include issues like choking or coughing when eating, aspiration pneumonia, low albumin protein the bloodstream, or bed sores. Also of note, PEGs can produce adverse reactions including infection, bleeding, or perforation (rupturing through the stomach). Some patients with dementia or confusion may also pull the PEG out since they do not remember why the PEG was placed in the first place. At present, years of research have led national medical societies to advise against placing PEG tubes in patients with advanced dementia and recommend the practice of "comfort feeding" or "pleasure feeding" instead.

At this juncture, we encourage our patients and family members to reframe the thinking. Your loved one is not dying because she's not eating. She is not eating because she's dying. It's certainly a difficult concept to entertain, but one worth pondering and discussing.

Food

NPO, DIET COKE, AND ORANGE SODA

On the other hand, there are situations where the patient really wants to eat but has a stomach or intestinal obstruction or has suffered a stroke and cannot swallow or process food. In these cases, medically, the patient would be made NPO. In some instances, the patient is awake and alert and really wants something to taste, yet their families, with the best of intentions, withhold food or drink from them because of the doctor's orders.

I still remember a young lady who had end-stage kidney failure but refused dialysis adamantly, and even pulled out multiple dialysis catheters. All she wanted every time I visited her hospital room was a Diet Coke!

I can remember another elderly woman who had intestinal obstruction. She was in the intensive care unit (ICU) and was high risk for surgery. The plan was to wait things out and see if her obstruction would resolve itself. She persistently requested orange soda, but of course, she was NPO. The ICU team was very worried that she would not be able to keep the soda down and would throw it up. I was called to provide a palliative care consult to help resolve some of these issues for the patient and aid the ICU team.

While I understood that she certainly could not drink a whole bottle of soda and would certainly vomit and become very uncomfortable, what about one sip? What about just gurgling the orange soda in her mouth for taste and to get that carbonated zing?

The patient looked at me longingly. I proposed this to the ICU doctor and nurse. "How about we dip a mouth swab in orange soda and swab her mouth? That would make the patient more comfortable and happier, and she wouldn't really swallow any significant amount." The ICU doctor and nurse looked at each other and nodded. I said, "Well, the only problem now is that we don't have orange soda."

With lightning speed, the patient's daughter pulled out a beautiful bottle of orange soda. "I have it. I had it all along in my bag. I was hiding it so no one would take it away from me."

The nurse went to get some swabs. We dipped the swab in the orange soda and the daughter lovingly swabbed her mom's mouth. I have never seen a more satisfied, toothless smile, or a happier ICU patient!

What this experience taught me was to not fight about it. Fighting makes everyone exhausted and stressed, including the patient. A great strategy is to reset our expectations and think outside the box.

COMFORT FEEDING

So, what's comfort or pleasure feeding? This term means you allow the patient to continue to eat and drink by mouth despite the risk that doing so might cause a chest infection or pneumonia. It means <u>acknowledging</u> and <u>accepting</u> the risk that feeding problems can happen at any time despite our best collective efforts. Because of these factors, sometimes it's best to allow the patient the pleasure of tasting foods that they like.

Depending on the situation, it may be best to stop any dietary restrictions like low-salt or low-sugar diets and let the patient eat whatever they want. This allows them to taste their favorite foods again! Of course, it's important to keep in mind that a resetting of expectations will be needed, as the patient will not be able to eat a whole plate of food. Small plates or tapas-sized foods will be offered instead to minimize adverse reactions.

In my experience with advanced dementia or cancer patients, many of them will eat very slowly—and sometimes only two to five spoonfuls during a meal. The important thing to remember is to create a pleasant environment—perhaps with nice music, flowers, and good company (family and friends)—and to always have a lot of patience.

Families should speak with doctors, nurses, dietitians, and speech/swallow therapists to learn the best and safest way to feed their loved ones. The top 10 tips I recommend include:

1. Only feed the patients when they are awake and alert.
2. Make sure the patient is sitting up or propped up in bed.

3. Always tilt the head forward.
4. Feed very slowly.
5. Use very small spoons (like baby spoons).
6. Offer their favorite foods in very small amounts.
7. Monitor their throats and ensure you see swallowing movements.
8. Check their mouths to see if there's any leftover food (a.k.a. "pocketing" food).
9. Clean their mouths at the end to remove any leftover food bits to prevent aspiration, which can lead to pneumonia.
10. Do not expect them to finish their plate/bowl.

*Bonus tip: Play some nice music while they eat!

If we don't do these things, we run the risk of fighting with our loved ones during each meal. This causes stress for ourselves and feelings of guilt that we are not doing enough. We may also risk losing precious time while we fight this losing battle. Instead of focusing on things that we cannot control, it's better to enjoy the time we have left. Consider this: If our loved one's time is limited, how do we want to spend that time? Fighting about food, or enjoying food at their speed and pace?

COFFEE AND CAKES

One day as I was driving around the tree-lined streets of Queens, I thought about how I should go about speaking with a patient of mine named Mr. Picalli. What could he be thinking about? Was he suffering? Did he have a lot of symptoms? Was he depressed, as many heart-failure patients are? What was I going to say to him? How should I respond to him?

Earlier that day, my hospice nurse manager urged me to give it a shot. "You better go see him. He just came onto hospice, and he's asking for physician-assisted suicide." Mr. Picalli was an elderly Italian man with end-stage heart failure.

I took a deep breath. Why couldn't this be an easy day?

Before I knew it, I was lost. It was before the age of Waze and effective GPS systems. All I had was a pre-printed Map Quest page with step-by-step directions that I had somehow suddenly misplaced.

Gathering myself and my thoughts, I focused on the direction I was going, appreciating the neighborhood

Food

stores that represented the great immigrant diversity of Queens. I turned onto his street and found parking easily right in his driveway—a rarity in some parts of Queens. I opened my trunk and took out my doctor's bag. When I knocked on his door, an elderly lady in a sunny yellow dress and an apron with a bright red tomato on it greeted me.

As I stepped inside the house, the comforting aroma of freshly made coffee enveloped my senses. I walked through the living room and placed my doctor's bag on one of the chairs in the dining room. Mrs. Picalli motioned me to go into the bedroom where Mr. Picalli was sitting in his wheelchair. He had just bathed and shaved, and the smell of shaving cream was still in the air.

"Good morning, Mr. Picalli. How are you doing today?"

"All right, I guess. What's your name?"

"My name is Dr. Pan, and I am visiting you from hospice."

"Can you give me a shot to end it all?"

"Mr. Picalli, this is a heavy request. Can you tell me what you're thinking about?"

"They told me in the hospital that this is it. There's no cure, no treatment for me. I might as well get it over with. What's the point?"

"I can see that this is a very difficult time for you."

"Yeah. So, about the shot. Do you think you can do it?"

"I'm not sure, Mr. Picalli. What else did they tell you in the hospital? What else have you been thinking about?"

"Well, they told me it's only a matter of time. I don't want to sit around and wait. My poor wife—she gets so nervous."

"Maybe we can ask your wife to come in so we can talk together?"

"All right. I guess we can go to the dining room and talk to her. Can you wheel me out?"

In the dining room, Mrs. Picalli sat clasping her hands around a coffee mug, her fingers fidgeting and

Food

tapping around the mug. I wheeled Mr. Picalli to the dining table and locked the wheelchair brakes.

This time, the aroma of cake baking in the oven distracted me.

"Wow, what smells so good?" I asked.

"When I get nervous, I bake. I cook. Nowadays, I'm doing lots of cooking and baking!" exclaimed Mrs. Picalli. "But he has no appetite. He doesn't eat like he used to."

"I just don't have the appetite anymore. I can't eat. I can't sleep. I just keep thinking about the end."

"Sounds like you may be experiencing some anxiety or depression, Mr. Picalli," I explored. "A lot of people who have advanced heart disease get anxious or depressed. If we treat these symptoms, you may feel better. What do you think about that?"

"Sure, I'll try it. It's either that or taking the shot."

"Can we not talk about the shot anymore? It's making me very nervous. Anyone want a piece of cake? I just baked a carrot cake. It's my mother's recipe. Doctor, would you like some coffee and cake?" Mrs. Picalli stood up to head to the kitchen.

"Sure, Mrs. Picalli. I would love some cake and coffee. While you get that, I will talk to your husband some more, all right?"

Mr. Picalli listened intently as I explained to him the medication I wanted to prescribe for him to treat his anxiety/depression. I also told him it might be a good idea for the hospice social worker and chaplain to come for a visit, and they could offer him further emotional and spiritual support. As it turned out, he was eager for help.

When his wife came out with a tray of cake and coffee, Mr. Picalli actually ate a small piece. It made his wife very happy.

I wound up visiting Mr. Picalli multiple times and we became good friends. He responded to treatment for his anxiety and depression, and we were able to stabilize his cardiac symptoms. He began walking again, slowly, and in the house only. But that was much better than sitting in the wheelchair all day.

Food

Every time I visited, Mrs. Picalli always made sure we had fresh coffee and her best cake recipes. Chocolate cake. Strawberry shortcake. Carrot cake. Rainbow cookies. Apple pies. À la mode. With so many tasty options, it's no wonder their house was one that I always looked forward to visiting!

After a few conversations, there were no more talk of "shots." At our hospice interdisciplinary team meetings, Mr. Picalli was a success story!

Ten months later, Mr. Picalli was thriving. Because he was doing so well, I now had to tell him that he was "graduating" from hospice! Although rare, hospice graduations do happen from time to time. It was a bittersweet event. The good news was he was no longer dying or declining. On the other hand, we had to part ways, and he would be discharged from hospice services. This was bad news for us, as we had become good friends. In the end I was the one grieving—not because my patient died, but because he lived.

LESSONS

- When a loved one has an advanced illness, it's very common for them to lose their appetite and a decent amount of weight. Another way to reframe this is they're not dying because they are not eating; they are not eating because they are dying.
- Work with your doctor to make sure reversible causes are treated. These may include constipation, oral thrush, depression, pain, lack of social company, and ill-fitting dentures.
- A great strategy is to *reset* our expectations and use "comfort" or "pleasure feeding" strategies to focus on enjoying each other's company!
- Another great strategy to consider is to ask your doctor and medical team to review all your medications, and "deprescribe" whatever pills that may not be necessary for end-of-life care! Too many pills and meds may create side effects and contribute to anorexia as well.

BREAK FOR A FAVOR!

If you are enjoying this book,
please write a brief positive review on the
platform where you bought this book.

Bonus Favor: Would you please leave
a photo with your review?

Extra Bonus Favor: Could you please leave
a video review to make extra impact?

Thank you in advance!

I truly appreciate your help!

CHAPTER 4

Music at the End of Life

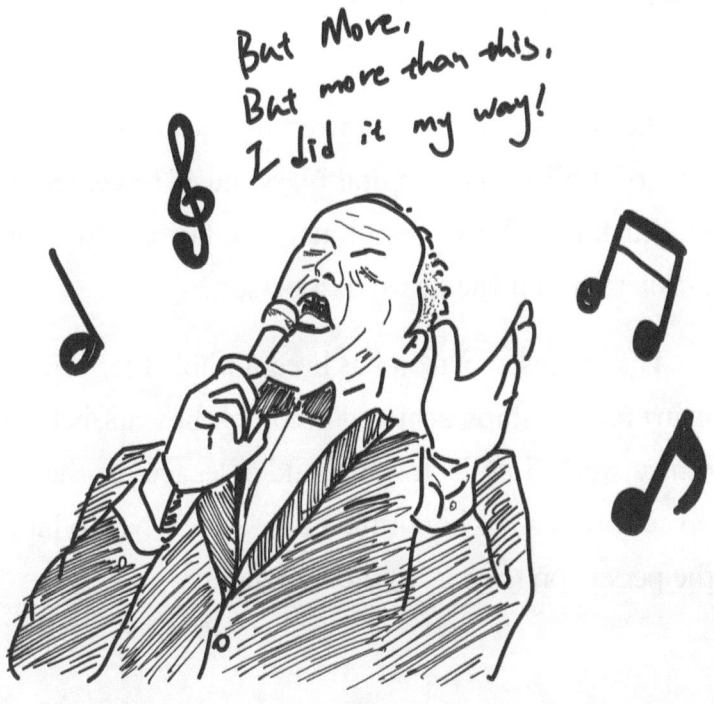

AT THE HOSPITAL WHERE I WORK, WHEN A BABY'S born, the father pulls on a chain by the bedside, and a lullaby plays overhead throughout the whole hospital.

We can be in the middle of a team meeting, a conference, or a patient interview, and all of a sudden, the "Brahms' Lullaby" goes off. We stop our conversations, listen, and take a moment to reflect on the baby, this new life, and the promise of hope and future that he or she could achieve! Alternatively, we get annoyed by the interruption to our normal workflow.

But at some point, I started to question the fairness of it all. If the hospital plays music to celebrate the birth of a person, wouldn't it be fair to also play music to honor the death of a person?

The deceased person has lived a whole life, formed many relationships, achieved accomplishments, helped others, worked, and left some kind of legacy. Yet, there's no celebration, no honoring—only a body bag to hide the person on the way to the morgue.

SONGS TO CELEBRATE A LIFE

I had some fun thinking about what song should be played over the loudspeakers to celebrate a life and received input from my patients. Here are a few we thought would be fitting:

- "My Way" by Frank Sinatra
- "Another One Bites the Dust" by Queen
- "Stairway to Heaven" by Led Zeppelin
- "For He's a Jolly Good Fellow," a French melody
- "Hallelujah" by Jeff Buckley

I took my research further on YouTube. I searched for popular songs about death and dying or that are popular at funeral services. Many wonderful, amazing songs came up. Some I was familiar with, like "Somewhere Over the Rainbow" by Israel Kamakawiwo'Ole, "Live Like You Were Dying" by Tim McGraw, "I've Had the Time of My Life" by Bill Medley and Jennifer Warnes, and "Forever Young" by Rod Stewart.

I learned of other songs that are wonderful as well, like "I'll Be Seeing You" by Billie Holiday, "The Dance" by Garth Brooks, "See You Again" by Wiz Khalifa, "You Can Close Your Eyes" by James Taylor, "Follow the Sun" by Xavier Rudd, "I'll Be Missing You" by Puff

Daddy and Faith Evans, and "Prop Me Up Beside the Jukebox (If I Die)" by Joe Diffie.

My number one favorite would be "My Way" by Frank Sinatra! Hands down. I identify with the song's message. Apparently, I'm not the only one. In my experience with dying patients and their families, whenever I have asked them if they would like me to play a song for them, "My Way" was the song that was often requested. I would sit down, take out my iPhone, and play the beautiful, reflective song.

AND NOW, THE END IS NEAR...

Music often comes into play with palliative extubations, which is when you disconnect someone from the ventilator for life support based on the patient's and family's wishes. When patients are dying, the ventilator may not be providing "life support" anymore and is instead becoming a "death-prolonging" intervention. Regardless, it's a very emotional time, and you never really know how long the patient is going to survive after the disconnection from the ventilator—although generally, it's longer than you might think. More about that later.

Relatives in that moment want to do something. They might want to feed their loved one, for instance, but if somebody's unconscious, you can't feed them. That often brings us to music, and finding their favorite song or something that's applicable for the moment.

On a wintery evening, I was caring for an elderly Latina woman whose lungs, heart, and kidney functions all began to give out. Despite the ventilator and attempts at life support, her condition was quickly deteriorating. I had a long conversation with her husband and other family members. They said she was a proud and independent woman, the "matriarch" of the family. She would never want to linger like this. They decided to remove the life support tubes and machines and allow her to die naturally, preserving her dignity.

After we pre-medicated her, the tubes and machines were disconnected. She was peaceful, breathing on her own for the last minutes to hours of her life. The room was calm and at peace. I asked her husband if she had a favorite song she would want us to play. Without hesitation, he said, "A ella le encanta, 'De Mi Manera!'" (she loves "My Way").

As I translated the words into English in my head, "De Mi Manera" sounded very much like "My Way." But could this be the same song? Or a different Spanish song that I knew nothing about? So I asked him, "Es una cancion Espanola?" ("Is this a Spanish song?")

He said, in such a righteous and Spanish way, "No, es *Frank Sinatra*!"

DANCING THE ARTHRITIS MACARENA

Mrs. P.R. was a 68-year-old Latina woman who was hospitalized for respiratory failure from multiple conditions. Despite many doctors and nurses advising her that she had to use her BIPAP oxygen mask (which was a kind of non-invasive respirator), she chose not to wear it. She consistently complained it was too tight and uncomfortable for her. Mrs. P.R. told many of us, "Whenever God is ready for me, I am ready to go." She knew what she was talking about, since she had already been intubated and artificially maintained on the ventilator twice before. Hearing this, we called Mrs. P.R.'s husband to notify him of her decision. He sounded burdened and sad but acknowledged that he knew about her wishes and would respect them. He wanted to come to the hospital to talk to her one more time, to convince her to "cooperate with the doctors." We arranged to meet up with him and talk to her together.

I, along with our social worker, met with Mrs. P.R.'s husband outside her room. His name was Luis. Unlike the elderly, kyphotic man that we conjured based on the phone call, Luis dressed like a biker, sporting a leather jacket and a bandana on his head. He huffed and puffed, telling us "I can't deal with her no more. I got my own problems. I got COPD, I got back problems—I can't even work out no more." He pointed to his right and left shoulders, both sides of his back, his right and left hips, saying, "I got pain here, here, here and here."

The way he moved reminded me of a dance, and I couldn't help but remark to him. "You look like you are doing the arthritis macarena!" He stared at me, then we all burst out laughing in the middle of the hospital hallway.

LESSONS

- Enjoy music at every stage of life, including at the end of life. Bringing some music into these moments can really help!
- Music transcends cultures. Explore some different songs from different countries and cultures!
- Even amidst challenges and serious conversations, find some time for dance moves and humor!
- Have you picked out your "end-of-life theme song?"

CHAPTER 5:

Family Meetings

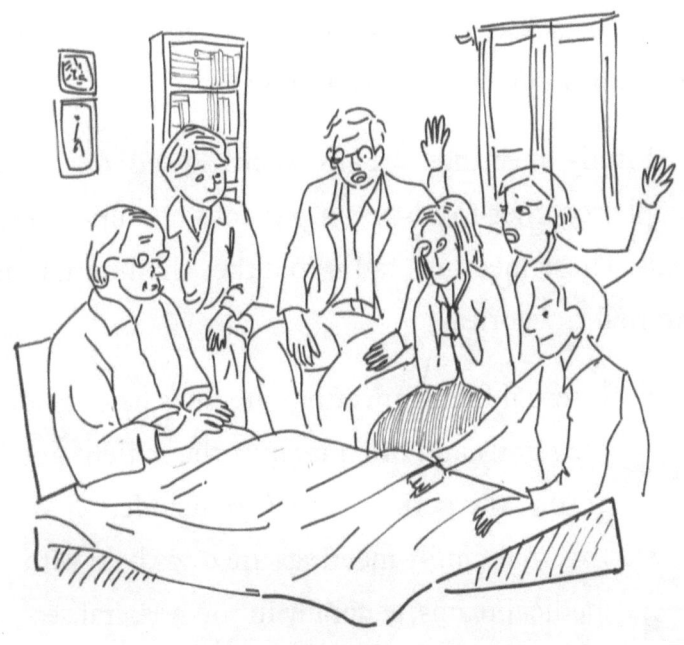

LET'S TALK ABOUT FAMILY.

Families need to be able to get together and support each other when a loved one is facing end of life.

I know—that may be easier said than done!

Relatives who may not talk to each other, let alone have a good relationship, could find themselves forced to collaborate in order to decide care options for a relative for which they may have complicated feelings. Or they may find themselves unsure of what to do—wracked with guilt, anger, or sadness over the decision they're being asked to make.

Family meetings are frequently used to bring people together to discuss a patient's condition and goals. These meetings fall into either the internal or external categories:

- Internal family meetings are ones held inside the family and often include the patient and anyone the patient wishes to include.
- External family meetings are ones held with medical teams, generally in the hospital setting. This is especially true when geriatrics or palliative care teams are involved and are used to ensure everyone's voice is heard, concerns are presented, and questions are answered. Remembering that this is about

the patient and not about individual concerns of family members is important, and the goal here is to make a plan that everyone can support.

THE IMPORTANCE OF BEING HEARD

Family meetings are very important to bring everybody together and get them on the same page. They are also needed to make sure that everybody who has something to say gets the chance to be heard.

Otherwise, the person who is the proxy, the mouthpiece, or the decision-maker often ends up getting blamed. Why did you do this? Do you love him? Do you care? You only want to save money! You only want his or her money! You never called or consulted with us!

It's very easy to play Monday morning quarterback and blame someone for making decisions. That's why it's important to have family meetings where everyone is heard and their concerns are voiced.

The decision-makers are tasked with very difficult choices—and typically, at the behest of the medical team. Their role is to put themselves in the patient's shoes—decide what the patient would want. It helps when the patient has a living will or some evidence of their thoughts. Remember, this isn't about what the relatives want, it's what the patient wants.

When we meet with family, we instruct them that we need everyone to support the decision-makers and not blame them. We say that very transparently. Ahead of family meetings, I also try to align and pre-meet with the other medical specialties to make sure we're all on the same page—we cannot be telling people different things. If we get our message crossed, it's game over. The family won't ever trust us.

As a patient or a family member, it's important to learn skills on how to talk to your doctors. You can ask your doctors to tell you the truth in a supportive way. If you have multiple doctors or specialists, you can ask them to conference with each other and come up with a unified plan and present it to you.

Family Meetings

FIGHT-OR-FLIGHT MODE

When you're faced with a crisis, it's common to enter fight-or-flight mode. Fighting may mean getting angry and walking out. Flight may mean failing to show up or answer calls—denial or avoidance.

Fight-or-flight mode comes into play sometimes during family meetings—and when someone is in this state, they're not really rational or able to absorb information. As a result, we try to use different team members—whether that's chaplains, social workers, or others, in addition to doctors and nurses—to try and help relatives to emotionally process the situation and return to a calm state.

There are things that you can do to help keep calm while you digest and face this unsettling news. Here are a few of my go-to recommendations:

- The most effective way to return to that calm state is also the simplest—just breathe. You can try box breathing like this: breathe in for four seconds, hold for four seconds, breathe

out for four seconds, and hold for four seconds. Repeat four times.
- Try not to jump ahead too much! Take things one step and one day at a time. When everything piles up, it often becomes overwhelming.
- Don't be afraid to ask questions to clarify the situation. There are no stupid questions.
- Another option to consider is dialectical behavioral therapy,[2] or DBT. It's used for mindfulness practice, emotional regulation, and crisis management.
- Get in your push-ups and sit-ups! Intense exercise can leave you in a better mental state.

DEREK THE "JACK-OF-ALL-TRADES"

Derek was a contractor who handled many large projects, and the results always came out amazing. While some contractors focused on carpentry or electric, Derek knew quite a bit about all the trades. His

---

[2] "Dialectical Behavior Therapy (DBT)," Cleveland Clinic, last reviewed April 19, 2022, https://my.clevelandclinic.org/health/treatments/22838-dialectical-behavior-therapy-dbt.

family and friends called him "jack-of-all-trades" or the "Renaissance man." He was the patriarch of his family and had five children. He adored all of them and they loved him for who he was. Derek taught his three boys and two girls to be physically, emotionally, and financially independent. All of his children followed his advice to achieve careers that they enjoyed. His son Adam was a lawyer, daughter Betty a doctor, son Craig a carpenter, son David an accountant, and daughter Evelyn an artist. Derek and I agreed how amazing it was that children can be raised in the same family yet be so different and have different skill sets.

As Derek became ill with chronic comorbid conditions that made him more and more frail, we talked about him holding a family meeting to discuss things openly and frankly. Rather than placing all the responsibilities on one or two people, I suggested giving everyone a chance to shine. This would be accomplished by allowing each person to take responsibility by using their individual strength to do something they are good at! I guided Derek on how to conduct this type of conversation, gave his children a heads up, and set expectations for attendance and participation.

After pondering about the family meeting for some time, Derek decided he would try it. I explained to Derek that this was *not* about placing a burden on his children. This was about open communication and should be seen as an opportunity for them to ask questions so his children would be able to help out and feel useful. We reviewed the steps again and he called the meeting. He was nervous, but he knew he had to do it.

On the day of the meeting, he ordered some food and snacks and played some oldies music they all enjoyed—again, food and music playing a role. Derek told his children about his compounding medical conditions and that he wanted to be open with his family. He didn't want there to be any secrets. Adam acknowledged how important it was to get the family together and volunteered to help with legal matters such as wills, living wills, power of attorney, and healthcare proxy appointments. Betty chimed in to help with healthcare proxy matters, to accompany Derek to his doctors' appointments, and to be the person who would learn more about his treatment plans. Craig volunteered to build a ramp in the backyard so that Derek could use his wheelchair if he wished. David offered to help with financial matters, paying bills, and managing the tax season. Evelyn offered to stop by more frequently to play music and cards with Derek and to take him out for fresh air when he wanted. The family meeting turned out exceptionally well, and they laughed and reminisced about old times. They all decided this was quite helpful and that they should meet once a month to touch base. Derek breathed a sigh of relief and felt supported by his family. No one felt burdened because everyone was chipping in, doing what they could and what they excelled at.

WHEN THINGS ARE MORE DIFFICULT

It's important to keep in mind that while the meeting above turned out to be simple and straightforward to organize, others are very, very difficult.

Exit Strategies

I get along well with most of my patients and their families—but every once and again, no matter what I do or say, I just know it's not going to work. In a challenging case, the family I was helping was very detail-oriented, which isn't necessarily a bad thing! We want relatives to be informed about what's going on.

But in this case, the relatives reached out to patient services because they said they weren't getting the answers they needed. It's a resource for patients and families with questions or concerns about their care.

"Maybe it's a good idea if you wrote down a list of the questions you have," a hospital rep told them. So they did. They put together a page full of cumbersome and detailed questions about the difference between palliative and hospice care, the options available to them, the venue for each care option, feeding and nutrition, hydration, and many others. They also wanted to know how all of these options would impact life expectancy, how to add breathing and ventilation options, and on, and on, and on.

The family was buried in minutiae—they were losing the forest for the trees.

Family Meetings

None of the details they wanted to ask about truly mattered, because ultimately, they didn't know what they wanted. We needed to resolve the bigger-picture issues first before dealing with everything else.

In these types of situations, when a relative is facing the prospect of end-of-life care, here's what I recommend:

- Make it a point to come together.
- Ask questions if you need to.
- Make a list of questions or concerns.
- Ask the medical teams to talk to each other and present a unified message.
- Ask for a palliative care consult.
- Ask for an organized family meeting.
- Do your best to consider what the *patient* would want and what would matter most to the patient.

MONA, THE "QUEEN OF SHOPPING"

Mona was in her late 60s, had retired from her accounting job, was living on her own, was not married, and had no kids. She was a chain smoker, and despite many conversations with her doctor, she continued to smoke. Although she had mounting COPD and heart disease, she was able to keep doing the things she loved, like getting her mani-pedi on a regular basis. Her friends dubbed her the "queen of shopping," as she loved to roam through shopping malls and to get the best deals. Mona landed in the hospital with infections in her urinary tract (UTI) and bloodstream (bacteremia). This led to sepsis and shock. Her blood pressure plummeted and her lungs stopped functioning properly. Since Mona did not have a spouse or children, her cousin Nicki stepped up to speak with her doctors.

According to Nicki, they were pretty close and sometimes went shopping together. Like many people, Mona did not have detailed advance directives. However, Nicki did remember a conversation where Mona had said she wanted to have CPR resuscitation. Nicki could not recall what the circumstances were or why Mona had that conversation with her. There were also no discussions about what would happen after the resuscitation if the outcome was not successful.

Family Meetings

At this point, Mona was in a stupor—her eyes would open but she could not really process complex information or make her own medical decisions. Nicki came to the hospital as much as she could to visit Mona and try to rouse her, but to no avail.

When I called Nicki up, she was tired, stressed, and lost. I acknowledged that this was a very emotional and exhausting time and that our palliative care team was consulted on Mona's case because Mona was seriously ill. I told Nicki that our goal was to support her through this tough time. Nicki confided that she felt guilty because she was not going to come in that day to see Mona. She was too fatigued and stressed and did not feel she was safe to drive.

As we spoke about Mona's situation and how sick she was, Nicki said the only thing she was pretty sure of was that Mona should be resuscitated but could not state any reasoning. Nicki also told us that Mona had a niece—a daughter of one her brothers who had passed away. Nicki called the niece and her immediate reaction was, "You should let her go peacefully. Don't let them put her on any machines. She wouldn't want that."

Exit Strategies

After that brief conversation, Nicki did not want to speak with the niece anymore. I strongly suggested a family meeting for Nicki and the niece to speak together with our palliative care and medical teams. The idea was to hear from all sides, all stakeholders, and put a complete picture together about what was happening with Mona. Nicki said she would think about it.

A couple of days passed—which is a lot of time in the hospital and ICU—and I did not hear back from Nicki. I spoke with the ICU and the ICU doctors said Mona was not responding to any treatment. As much as they tried to be hopeful and positive, they weren't optimistic that she would make it.

The ICU tried to call Nicki, but she stopped answering the team's calls. This left us in a tough spot.

In cases where the patient is not doing well, the medical teams have tried their best, and the family is not accessible to give updates or talk about next steps, we ask for an ethics consultation to discuss the case as a group. The intention is to figure out the right thing to do.

Family Meetings

We made another call to Nicki and left a message that we were asking for an ethics consult to discuss Mona's case because we were stuck. At that point—finally—Nicki called us back and agreed to a family meeting.

We held a virtual family meeting with Nicki, Mona's niece, our palliative care doctors, and our social worker. We talked about Mona's situation and explained that everything that could be done had been done, and Mona was not getting better. We acknowledged that Nicki was struggling with the resuscitation situation because of this casual conversation and focused on the goals of care moving forward. Again, the goal was to decide what would be truly meaningful for Mona.

Mona was at the end of her life. There was no reversing or curing her pre-existing heart disease and COPD (a.k.a. emphysema).

No matter what care she received, she would not be returning home or be able to go shopping again, and she would not be enjoying a future mani-pedi.

If we proceeded aggressively, we could surgically do a tracheostomy (cut a hole in her throat) and permanently connect Mona to life support machines, surgically place a feeding tube (PEG), and give her artificial feedings. Mona would then be shipped off to a nursing home for her remaining days.

Alternatively, we could refocus efforts to provide Mona with comfort-oriented care, compassionately remove her from invasive treatments like artificial life support tubes and machines and allow her to die a natural and peaceful death.

When Nicki and the niece talked things out together and remembered what Mona's life was like, they concluded that Mona would not really wish to linger on artificial support machines. Nicki and the niece reminisced about good times they spent, jokes they used to tell, and decided to compassionately remove the tubes and machines, giving Mona a dignified death.

We set up a date. Nicki came in for the compassionate extubation, kept Mona company, and held her hand. After the heavy ventilator equipment was removed from the room, we sat in Mona's hospital room with light jazz music playing—it was Mona's favorite. There was a feeling of peace and lightheartedness that reminded me of a light Sunday brunch. Nicki confided that the family meeting was very helpful, even though, at first, she was hesitant about it. As I told Nicki, it can be difficult for family members in these emotional situations to talk openly, be objective, and to not argue or blame each other. When emotions run high, people can get into the "fight-or-flight" mode. That's why we truly recommend family meetings facilitated by our palliative care or medical team members who are trained to mediate these conversations.

LESSONS

- Internal and external family meetings can help to ensure that everyone is aligned. Internal family meetings are ones held inside the family. This includes the patient and anyone the patient wishes to include. External family meetings are held with medical teams and generally take place in a hospital setting (especially when geriatrics or palliative care teams are involved)

to gather everyone's voice, hear concerns, and answer questions.
- Remember, family meetings are about the patient—and making a plan that everyone can support. Please be sure to use your palliative care team as a resource in helping your family get and stay on the same page.
- When emotions run high, take deep breaths, or splash some cold water on your face. Try to avoid "fight-or-flight" responses. Try not to run away. On the other hand, if you truly need more time, you can ask for the meeting to be rescheduled.

CHAPTER 6

Total Pain and the Vortex

A LOT OF PEOPLE WILL SAY "I DON'T REALLY FEAR dying; I fear being in pain."

When people have pain, they start to disengage and withdraw. They don't want to do this or that. And it can significantly diminish their quality of life.

Physical pain is easy to recognize, but there are lots of forms of pain. There's emotional pain, spiritual pain, social pain, existential pain, and financial pain. All of those various types of pain coalesce to define *total pain*—a palliative care concept codified by Dame Cecily Saunders, the founding mother of hospice in England.

PHYSICAL PAIN

Patients get moved to palliative care the moment they say they want to die or if they decline other care options because the pain is just too difficult for them to handle.

We recently had a patient on dialysis who started declining to go to his dialysis treatments. Palliative care was called in, and we visited with him.

"Mr. Smith, do you realize that you use dialysis because your kidneys don't work?" we asked.

"Yes," he said.

"Why don't you want to go to dialysis treatments?"

"Because when they lay me down in the dialysis chair and put me back, my leg hurts."

"If we treat your leg pain, would you go to dialysis?"

"Yes, yes."

That situation could have been resolved earlier with a simple conversation.

EMOTIONAL PAIN

We had a patient who is Burmese and was diagnosed with advanced cancer. At first he wanted to aggressively treat the cancer. But that didn't go well, and it came with lots of side effects.

Then his kidney function declined because the cancer was pressing on his kidney tubes.

He was offered dialysis and tried it, but that was very painful for him, and he chose not to continue. I went to visit him, and he was very gracious.

"Thank you for coming to see me. I'm very lonely," he told me. "My family is mad at me, and they deserted me."

"I didn't get the word that they deserted you. They're coming to see you, and we were just on the phone with them," I responded.

"They're mad at me."

"Why are they mad?"

"Because I yelled at them and said some mean things."

"Well, maybe you shouldn't yell at them. Maybe you should apologize."

"No, no, no. They know."

"Well, I'm gonna call them and tell them you apologized."

"I do feel really bad about yelling at them."

"I'm gonna tell them that you feel that."

"No, no, no. It's too late for that."

"All right," I told him (in my mind, I told myself, I'm totally calling them to say that he was sorry, but he didn't have the guts to say it himself). I continued. "You have to stop yelling at your family. They're really trying to help you. And on the other hand, you're lonely. It's not that they don't care about you. They're afraid to come see you because you yell at them."

"Okay," he said.

Later, we called his family and told them he felt really bad, and the family also showed remorse.

"We didn't think he would say that," they told us.

"We took it upon ourselves to say it because he couldn't, but he does feel bad," I said.

"Thank you for telling us. It means a lot," they said.

SPIRITUAL PAIN

Some patients feel existential or spiritual pain when they get a terminal diagnosis. They start to wonder, "Why did this happen to me? What did I do to deserve this illness? Why did God abandon me?"

If a patient or their family is facing emotional distress, whether they're crying, sad, angry, or anything else, they should call the hospital's chaplain for help.

When you meet with a doctor, there's always an agenda, whether for a procedure, consent, or to make a medical decision. For social workers or case managers, it's about getting out of the hospital. But for spiritual care, there's really no agenda. Chaplains are trained to listen and to help relieve a patient's suffering at many levels. I want to encourage you to ask for the chaplains and speak with them. Don't be afraid.

It's also important to note that chaplains or pastoral care representatives are *not* the same as church or religious leaders. Chaplains or pastoral care representatives may belong to a faith affiliation, but they are trained to support patients of all faiths, and they are trained to not proselytize.

FINANCIAL PAIN

I had a patient who was intubated and received a tracheostomy because he was not improving. He could write on a whiteboard, and the first thing he wrote centered around his financial obligations.

There he was, completely dependent on other people without the ability to breathe on his own, and he was worried about money.

MRS. ROAN

Mrs. Roan was an 88-year-old woman who came onto hospice with a roar. Immediately everyone knew about her. Her intestines were blocked by her ovarian cancer, and her venting stomach tube was leaking. Her pain was out of control. She was agitated and her private aide called for help. The nurse manager in the office called and asked if I could rearrange my schedule to see her as soon as possible.

I walked the hallway searching for Mrs. Roan's apartment number. She was located at the end of the hall, which meant she had a corner apartment. I rang the bell and a middle-aged, olive-skinned woman opened the door. "Hi. Are you Dr. Pan? My name is Dolly, Mrs. Roan's aide." From her accent I surmised she might be from Guyana. Dolly introduced me to another elderly woman with bright blonde hair. "This is Audrey, the housekeeper." We walked past a posh living room decorated with golden draperies and carpet and elegant Victorian sofas. Dolly introduced me to another woman. "This is Priscilla, the night time aide." We then proceeded to Mrs. Roan's bedroom. She was lying in a hospital bed, eyes closed, hair out of place. Dolly called to her and announced that the doctor was here.

Mrs. Roan opened her eyes. "Finally, a doctor comes."

I shook her hand.

"Hello, Mrs. Roan. I'm so glad to meet you. How is your day going?"

"Terrible," she grunted.

"What's bothering you?" I asked.

She rolled her eyes.

"Are you having pain?"

"Yes."

"Can you tell me where?"

"All over," she snapped.

I gently palpated her chest, abdomen, legs, and arms. Mrs. Roan took it well. No sign of significant grimace or tenderness. I asked her to lift her legs and arms, and she was able to do so, despite some weakness.

Something in my gut told me to explore. "Do you feel the pain is more physical or emotional?"

Total Pain and the Vortex

She glared at me. "What kind of question is that? What kind of doctor are you?" She pursued further. "Are you that ridiculous doctor from the hospital?"

"No, Mrs. Roan. We have never met before," I reassured her.

"Are you sure?"

"Yes, I would remember," I said, finding the humor in the situation.

"Okay." She rested.

"Mrs. Roan, are you feeling nauseated?" I continued with my history taking.

"Yes, terrible, all the time."

"How about nerves? Do you feel nervous or anxious?" I asked.

Mrs. Roan looked at me desperately. "Yes. Too many questions. You can't fix me."

"How about constipation? Do you feel constipated?"

"Yes, very constipated."

Dolly added, "Mrs. Roan has not had a bowel movement for almost two weeks."

"Ooooh. I need to do a rectal exam. Mrs. Roan, do you mind if I check you from below and do a rectal exam?" I asked.

"I guess so. But you won't get anything out of me." She grunted.

"Okay, but let's try." I motioned Dolly to help me turn Mrs. Roan to her side. I asked Audrey to bring over some chucks or towels. Dolly brought over disposable gloves and some Vaseline gel. I checked her rectum and began working on disimpacting the large amount of stool that I felt. "You have a lot of poop in there, Mrs. Roan. I'm going to take some out so you can feel better."

Dolly and Audrey stared in awe and reported to Mrs. Roan. "The doctor is taking out a lot. You have a lot in there."

"You've been very patient, Mrs. Roan. You're a real trooper," I said.

"Okay, that's enough," Mrs. Roan groaned.

"Okay, we're done. You did great," I agreed. Dolly and I helped her get into a comfortable position so she could rest.

I went over to the desk to review Mrs. Roan's medications. Dolly came over to help.

"How are you holding up, Dolly?" I asked.

"All right."

"How long have you been working with Mrs. Roan?" I explored.

"I've known her for about a year," Dolly continued. "Audrey has been here for about fifteen years."

"She's not an easy person to deal with, I can tell."

"You can say that again! Make sure you tell her family that," Dolly implored.

In between discussing her medications, Dolly filled me in on Mrs. Roan's family situation. She was never an easy person to get along with. She did not have many friends in the building even though she had lived there for years. She was widowed and had a son and a daughter. The son was behaving erratically, calling Mrs.

Roan all kinds of names over the phone. He demanded that she write him blank checks and would cash them for large amounts of money. At other times he would demand that she sell her stocks and transfer the funds to him. When she wouldn't, or couldn't, he would call her all sorts of names. Meanwhile, Mrs. Roan was in bed, confused, in pain, constipated, and nauseated. It turns out he was bipolar and not on medication. Her daughter, extremely successful by any measure, had not spoken with Mrs. Roan for many years. Apparently the family attorney had contacted the daughter about Mrs. Roan's condition but she has not called. Her granddaughter was now the closest relative to her and in charge of the situation.

I felt a wave of sadness as I absorbed the story. Here was Mrs. Roan, wealthy, living in a luxurious home. Yet, there was not much more I could say about her. Not loved, not surrounded by her family, not comfortable, and not in peace. She was suffering in multiple domains: physically, emotionally, socially, and spiritually.

Mrs. Roan was right. I could not "fix" her. No one could fix her. But I could help her. She was the poster child of the concept of *total pain*. She was suffering from not only physical pain, but also emotional, social, psychological, and spiritual pain.

Had I been trained strictly in a conventional medical mode, I would have felt powerless, like a failure. I could not save her life—she was dying. I could not fix her emotional life with years of family dynamics and complex relationships. I could not control her family and what they do. I could have let myself slide into the total pain syndrome of feeling guilty or helpless because I could not save or fix her.

But thanks to my years of geriatrics and palliative care training, I knew several things. One, this is not my vortex. I will not delve into this situation emotionally, because the "vortex" would chop me to pieces. Two, I had the ability to get her physical symptoms under control. Three, I had an excellent, interdisciplinary hospice team that could help address all the domains of suffering that she was experiencing. Not to "fix" her, but to help her express her feelings, review her life, and find opportunities for redemption and relief. At least she would not be completely isolated in her suffering. Even though her case was painful and suboptimal for me as a doctor, I chose not to suffer from it. I chose to reframe it into what I could control and what I could not. I did my best and was satisfied with that. At least a ray of sunshine could beam through the golden drapes from time to time.

Three days into her hospice stay, Mrs. Roan's physical symptoms were under good control. Her pain was down to a rating of "mild" and she did not have any side effects from the pain medication. Her constipation and nausea resolved. Our nurse called daily to make sure Dolly was supported and competent in giving the medications. Mrs. Roan became much nicer to her companions and to our hospice staff. Our social worker visited Mrs. Roan to help her process her feelings about her children. We all kept in touch with her granddaughter who felt much more reassured about her grandmother's situation. She knew who to call and what options there were should things not work out at home.

Mrs. Roan died a week later. Even though she was only on hospice for about three weeks, we were able to make her feel better and help her family. I am always amazed at how well we can get to know a person or a family in a short time. I suppose there's really no time to waste at the end of life.

A FAMILY'S PAIN AND SUFFERING

There's a Buddhist saying about pain and suffering: "Pain is inevitable, suffering is optional." This quote has been attributed to the Dalai Lama, Haruki Murakami, and M. Kathleen Casey. Identifying the first person to share this wisdom is less important than recognizing the inspirational nugget at the core of this simple mantra.

We all deal with pain.

Pain is what happens. It's like a terminal illness you didn't ask for.

Suffering is what the pain does to you—something you alone can control.

I was reminded of that saying after working with a patient who had a massive stroke. He had every possible intervention but just didn't wake up. And he wasn't getting better.

Then, his brain bleed started again.

We had a family meeting with his wife who was beside herself, wishing they had spent more time together.

The pain was that the patient is dying, and the suffering was his loved one blaming herself.

Their daughters helped to put things into perspective.

"Dad is a strong guy, and when he was previously using a walker, he was miserable—he had lost his pride. He doesn't want this," they said. "If he could wake up from this, he would be furious at us for keeping him alive like this."

They eventually decided to take him off the ventilator—a difficult, tender decision—and the goal was for everything to be peaceful. We talked about how sometimes when you really love someone, you have to let them go.

We warned his family that after being taken off the ventilator, the timing is unpredictable. It could be minutes, it could be hours, it could be days. It's just not up to us anymore. It's up to God or some type of higher force. The most important thing is being there and knowing that you did your best to preserve his dignity, because having all these tubes jutting out of his body when his prognosis was so poor wasn't something the patient would have wanted.

The relatives all came together, and his wife was able to find peace in that decision. The patient died three hours later.

Everybody was, of course, very sad.

"Let's remember that he had a great life," I counseled them. "He helped so many people and has a wonderful family—as is evidenced by all of you being here, supporting each other, telling us about him, and seeing how much you care about him. We should really celebrate his life and the legacy that lives through you."

LESSONS

- Pain and suffering have many dimensions. Think of the *total pain* concept when approaching someone who is seriously ill and how we can help them in different dimensions: physical, psychological, social, financial, and spiritual.

- Engage the medical and interdisciplinary team to help address each domain of the total pain syndrome.
- Pain is inevitable. Suffering is optional. For you, this could mean "don't jump into the vortex!" In life, painful events will happen. We cannot control them. What we *can* control is how we respond. We do not need to let the pain cause us to suffer. We can be our bigger selves, not blame or judge. Just let go and move on.

CHAPTER 7

Hospice

When people hear the term hospice, they think of being sent to a hospice facility. But these days, it's more common for people to receive home hospice care than it is inpatient hospice care at a nursing or assisted living facility.

People facing the end of their life often believe there's no way they could go home. They're dependent on staff and treatments and a hospital bed. They don't even consider home-based hospice care.

When I tell people about it, like the wife of the patient with end-stage liver cancer I highlighted earlier, they react with surprise.

"Wow, really? I can go home?" they ask.

With hospice—for those facing a prognosis of six months or less to live—all you need is a clear corner of your house with an electrical outlet and enough space for a bed, oxygen tank, and other medical supplies. Wheelchairs and other equipment can also be provided. Hospice care insurance usually covers much of the equipment, too.

Sometimes, for expediency, healthcare providers and case managers are quick to send patients to nursing homes and rehabilitation facilities, but that other option is regularly kept out of the conversation.

A WIDER RANGE OF CARE WITHOUT THE QUESTIONS

Notably, hospice can open up a wider range of medical care options.

Regular Medicare patients, for example, must meet certain oxygen saturation criteria to receive oxygen at home.

If you're on hospice care, there's no requirement—you can receive oxygen if you're short of breath without having to worry about the oxygen saturation numbers.

HOLDING FIRM

I was trying to help a patient's family get her uncle home, and his niece was encountering all sorts of barriers. The uncle didn't have a wife or children and needed a 24/7 aide to take care of him. He had dementia and was in the hospital for end-stage kidney disease.

The patient's niece didn't want him to continue with dialysis because her uncle really couldn't even understand what was happening. His quality of life was being significantly diminished. In the past, he'd been sent to a rehab facility, but all he wanted was to go home—home was the place that felt comfortable and familiar to him.

Typically, a patient like this would be sent to a nursing home, and his niece was facing pressure to continue with medical care while considering her uncle's wishes.

"I don't want him to go to a nursing home because he's going to get confused. He already has dementia. He won't know anybody. He won't know where he is.

Exit Strategies

And he's going to start getting agitated and belligerent. It won't be good for him or anyone else. Why can't he just go home?" she asked.

"You're absolutely right. And I'm going to do whatever I can to help you get home. There's no reason to try to push him somewhere else," I told her.

In a case like this, the patient wanted to go home, and it seemed like the best thing for them. It was entirely reasonable to make this happen. Even though it took a few more days, we coordinated with the medical team and social worker and discharged him home. It's true when they say, "There is no place like home."

THE LITTLE THINGS

People in hospice are a lot franker about their feelings.

You also get to see what's possible in the home environment with the patients rather than a more clinical setting. When people are sick, they typically want to be home because home represents freedom.

A patient in a nursing home or a hospital has to deal with the hospital or nursing home's schedule. If you press the bell to go to the bathroom, you might not get a fast response. You have to wait. At home, you can just get up whenever you want to go to the bathroom. If you want to eat a sweet snack and you're diabetic, so be it! If you're at the hospital and want to eat that cookie, good luck.

Sometimes it really comes down to the little things. And the little things—the little moments of freedom—can mean so much, especially if you're facing end of life.

THE IMPACT OF FAMILY

Hospice and home health aides are truly doing God's work. There's a huge market today for this type of work, especially following the COVID-19 pandemic and "The Great Resignation."[3] Beginning in early 2021 in the wake of the COVID-19 pandemic, "The

---

[3] Alexander Serenko, "The Great Resignation: The Great Knowledge Exodus or the Onset of the Great Knowledge Revolution?," *Journal of Knowledge Management* 27, no. 4 (2023): 1042–1055, https://doi.org/10.1108/JKM-12-2021-0920.

Big Quit" is an ongoing economic trend in which employees have voluntarily resigned from their jobs en masse. Many states even have programs where family members can apply to become aides to work with their relatives.

WHO SAYS YOU CAN'T GO HOME?

It's important to understand the full range of palliative care options available—including home hospice. While people who receive hospice care are facing the end of their life, many wind up living on hospice for many months. That was the case with former president Jimmy Carter, who announced he was receiving hospice care in February of 2023 and remained alive a year later, enjoying ice cream and staying in good spirits throughout.

Hospice care doesn't always mean someone is done fighting their illness—it can be refocusing on care that involves a balance of pain management, symptom control, and quality of life.

For many people, going home is all they want. And it could be the right option for you and your loved one, too.

LESSONS

- People facing the end of their life often believe there's no way they could go home. But through hospice, they can.
- Hospice can open up a wider range of supportive care.
- Hospice care doesn't mean someone is done fighting their illness! It's about re-directing care to involve a balance of pain management, symptom control, and quality of life.

CHAPTER 8

Terri Schiavo—A Missed Opportunity for Advance Directives

THE IMPORTANCE OF ADVANCE DIRECTIVES become crystal clear when considering the Terri Schiavo ordeal.[4]

Schiavo went into cardiac arrest at her Florida home in 1990 when she was 26 years old. The cardiac arrest was caused by hypokalemia induced by an eating disorder. She was resuscitated and revived but had extensive brain damage. She could not speak or eat by herself. A feeding tube was placed to give her artificial nutrition.

She underwent physical therapy, speech therapy, deep brain stimulation, and nerve stimulation. But

---

[4] C. Chistopher Hook and Paul S. Mueller, "The Terri Schiavo Saga: The Making of a Tragedy and Lessons Learned," *Mayo Clinic Proceedings* 80, no 11 (2005): 1449–1460, https://doi.org/10.4065/80.11.1449.

after years of effort, she was deemed by neurologists to be in a persistent vegetative state (PVS).[5] This is different from a coma where the person is asleep and has their eyes closed all the time. PVS is a state that can be described as "the lights are on, but nobody is home." The sleep-wake cycle is intact. The patient goes to sleep at night and wakes up in the morning. Terri would be awake in the daytime but often looking around in an aimless manner.

Her husband Michael—who'd been appointed her legal guardian—filed a petition to remove her feeding tube, as he believed that she would not have wanted to continue artificial life support to maintain her in PVS. Her parents opposed, and without a living will, legal challenges back and forth continued for seven years. Both sides continued to argue that they had her best interests. Congress and President George W. Bush even got involved. But the truth is, no one knew Terri's wishes, because she never expressed them.

---

5   Lily Guo, "Persistent Vegetative State," Osmosis from Elsevier, last modified August 25, 2022, https://www.osmosis.org/answers/persistent-vegetative-state.

Terri Schiavo—A Missed Opportunity for Advance Directives

Schiavo's feeding tube was finally removed in March of 2005, and she died in hospice care 15 years after her cardiac episode. If she had established and shared her advanced directives with her loved ones, they all could have avoided years of strife and struggle.

At the time that was happening, I talked to a lot of people about it, and it was 50/50—half of the people that I talked to supported pulling her artificial feeding tube, and the other half believed doing so amounted to murder. It's a very personal decision, and it's better for you to make that decision yourself than leave it up to loved ones who may not know your actual wishes.

This case, while tragic, spurred a national conversation about the importance of personal advance directives. Remember, *it always seems too early until it's too late.* We cannot wait for the last minute to hold these crucial conversations. As a doctor, I have seen this play out thousands of times.

I've used Terri's case to teach medical students, residents, and doctors-in-training. I remember in one class with medical students, I was discussing advance directives with them. These are all healthy, vibrant, young people, studying medicine and eager to become physicians. We talked about the possibility that what if something like Terri's situation happened to them. What would they do? What would they want? What would they tell their loved ones in advance about what to do for them? Here are some responses:

- "Just pull the plug now. This is not living."
- "I would want to do a trial of two weeks."
- "I would want to do a trial of at least one year. You are not PVS until one year of this neurologic status."
- "I will leave it to my parents."
- "I would want to leave it to my boyfriend. I'm gay and my parents don't even know."
- "I would want to a trial of twenty-seven years."
- "I don't want to talk about it, and *you can't force me.*"

Advance directives can be very hard to discuss, and some people cannot bring themselves to go there. But many can and will.

LESSONS

- Many people have preferences as it concerns their care at end of life, but never had a chance to express them. These decisions and preferences are deeply personal. Even your close family members and loved ones may not know how you feel. Be courageous and kind enough to tell them!
- It's never too early to talk about advance directives, and famous cases like Terri Schiavo's can help you to start conversations with your friends and families about what truly matters to you.
- By expressing your wishes about end-of-life care fearlessly and clearly, you can help relieve burdens and guilt from your loved ones and give them the gift of knowing what you want to do about your health, illness, and end stage of life.

CHAPTER 9

Religion and Spirituality

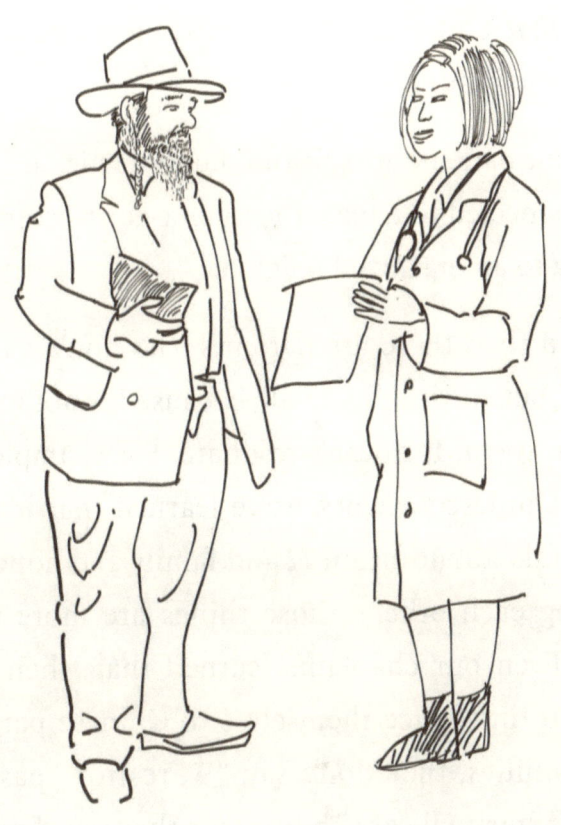

FAITH AND SPIRITUALITY ARE AMONG THE MOST sensitive topics we discuss with patients.

Some patients are so religious that they don't make medical decisions without the permission of the religious body. On the other hand, several of my Catholic patients said, "I'm Catholic, but I'm not really *that* Catholic." They seemed more ambivalent about their faith.

Some patients are spiritual, but not religious. They feel connected to a higher force but don't necessarily belong to an organized religion.

And then there are patients who don't want to talk about spirituality at all, because it's not important to them. It doesn't resonate. For example, for many Chinese patients, we've learned that it's better to talk about meaning and family and hope and helping each other—those things are more practical. Even our chaplains learned that when they come to introduce themselves to Chinese patients and families, they don't say, "We're from pastoral care or spiritual care," but rather they say, "You can think of me as a good friend who's had a lot of experiences in these things and who can really listen to your concerns and help you process what the doctors told you."

FICA

From a medical standpoint, there's a good tool for doctors to assess a patient's faith or spirituality, and the letters spell FICA:

- **Faith:** Do you have a faith affiliation? Is it spiritual or religious or some other kind of faith?
- **Involved:** If you have a faith community, how involved are you with your faith community? How big of a part of your life is it?
- **Community:** Is there a community that supports you? Is that community supportive, or does it pressure you?
- **Address:** As your doctor, how would you like me to address your faith concerns? I can talk with you more about it or not at all, or I can refer you to our chaplains.

For patients receiving end-of-life care and their loved ones, please make your comfort and interest discussing religion and spiritualty known! It's important for us to understand your spiritual needs so we can help you in the best way possible.

CHAPLAINS

When emotional and spiritual care are involved, we lean on our pastoral care chaplains.

My hospital's chaplains are excellent—they operate at a different dimension. Unfortunately, they're often called very late in a patient's life. Families and doctors usually think of calling them to give a patient last rites—but they want to interact with the patients and help them in their times of emotional need—not just at the very end.

Chaplains can be cross-denominational and are trained not to proselytize. So even if you believe in one religion, you don't have to have the chaplain from that religion to come and see you.

PRAYING FOR A MIRACLE

When things get tough, many relatives ask or pray for a miracle.

For a long time, those comments made me think, "They don't understand the gravity of the situation."

But then I went to a lecture by a chaplain, who said, "When people start talking about miracles, that means they understand. Because why else would they be asking for miracles?"

This is so true, and is such an amazing reframing that it helped me to reconsider my approach to patients and relatives who talk about miracles.

Often I'll ask my patients questions like, "What is a miracle to you? What does it look like? What does it sound like? What does it mean?" When they say "miracle," I might have an image of a miracle in my head—but is that the same image that they have?

Their miracle could be going home, or surviving for two months to meet their great-grandchild. It could involve making it to their next birthday. Until you share what that miracle is, it's impossible for your care team to know—and impossible for them to help you achieve it.

SOMETIMES MIRACLES DO HAPPEN!

Keep in mind that there are instances when patients of mine are facing end-of-life care and suddenly make a turnaround.

It does happen. Not all of the time, but sometimes. Maybe somebody has advanced gallbladder cancer and their skin was neon yellow from the bile building up. But after months of worry, surgery, and chemotherapy, they were able to recover, which is pretty amazing.

A recovery like that depends on the type of cancer, as well as the patient's overall health. The legendary cyclist Lance Armstrong, for example, is famous for recovering from testicular cancer—but not all cancers are the same. Somebody with pancreatic cancer won't have as high of a recovery rate. Certain types of lung cancer have different outlooks, too. Small-cell lung cancers are typically more responsive to chemotherapy, and the cancer often melts away. That's not the same for non-small-cell lung cancers.

When people talk about miracles, I usually tell them, "Let's hope for the best and have a plan B just in case." You never really know.

It's okay to think about miracles for you or your loved ones—and even better if you can define what a miracle is to you. Tapping into that can help you recognize what matters most and help you to define your care goals.

MEET MR. A, AN ELDERLY ORTHODOX JEWISH MAN

Mr. A was an 88-year-old Orthodox Jew with rheumatoid arthritis, hypothyroidism, and atrial fibrillation. He came to the Emergency Department (ED) after suffering a cardiac arrest at home. His son, Mr. B, found him unresponsive at home, called 911, and initiated CPR himself. Mr. A was resuscitated for 20 minutes, intubated by the paramedics, brought to the ED, went into asystolic cardiac arrest again, resuscitated for another 15 minutes, and brought back to life.

In the CCU, he developed ventricular tachycardia for which his son, always at the bedside, asked the medical team not to resuscitate him. He did not wish to sign any documents for "do not resuscitate" (DNR), as there was always a family member at the bedside to consult for such matters.

Mr. A's son requested that, in addition to his wife and sister, the family rabbi be consulted to help guide his decision-making. The palliative care team was consulted to assess goals and future care options.

The assumptions of the CCU were that because he was an Orthodox Jew, his family would want everything to be done, despite his very poor prognosis and the fact that he was dying. We held a family meeting that included the son and family, the palliative care doctors, the cardiology team, the hospital rabbi, and the family rabbi (by phone). After introductions, we asked Mr. B to summarize what he understood about his father's condition. He did so accurately, then emphasized that his father had made his wishes very clear. He did not want to be in pain, live in a vegetative state, or be a burden on anyone, and he wanted to "do it the Jewish way," abide by Jewish laws, principles, and ethics. Mr. B felt that he was being pressured to sign a DNR form and to make decisions about tracheostomy and feeding tube placement. He wanted more time to decide and asked what would happen if he refused to sign any papers or consents.

Given his knowledge of Jewish law, he needed time to clarify what would happen under the various treatment options being considered before providing consent for any procedure. At this point, we explained that we were not there to force him to make decisions. The issue at hand was how to decide on a treatment course that would address all of Mr. A's wishes.

One of Judaism's core tenets is that life has infinite value, and preserving it is of extreme importance. The Bible also teaches, concurrently, that death is inevitable. Jewish medical ethics help navigate these two seemingly contradictory teachings and are derived from Jewish religious law (Halacha). Basically, one is allowed to decline life-saving intervention if the interventions will only slightly delay the dying process, prolong or cause suffering, or are futile. Once an intervention is started, however, in general one cannot withdraw it with the expectation of death. This differs from biomedical ethical principles, which hold that there is no moral, ethical, or legal difference between withholding of life-sustaining treatments and withdrawing of such treatments, as long as the goals of care are clear.

After extensive discussion, the family rabbi clarified it would be acceptable to withdraw the patient from the ventilator if there were a "reasonable expectation" he would breathe on his own for a "reasonable amount of time." In this line of thought, if the patient's death were to occur, it would be part of the normal ventilator weaning process and not a direct and immediate consequence of the palliative extubation.

Following intermediation by the hospital rabbi, the definition of what would be a "reasonable expectation" and "reasonable amount of time" was established by the family rabbi as "over 50%" and "on the order of hours," respectively.

Subsequently, a pulmonologist was consulted to evaluate the possibility of weaning Mr. A from the ventilator. The pulmonologist concluded that the patient would likely be able to breathe for several hours after extubation, meeting the criteria outlined in the family meeting. As a result, Mr. A underwent palliative extubation. At 12 hours after the procedure, he died comfortably and naturally, surrounded by his family. His family was grateful for this outcome and for the hospital teams working with them.

MEET MR. J, A JAMAICAN MAN WITH HIS OWN BELIEFS AND "NEAR DEATH AWARENESS"

Mr. J, a 68-year-old Jamaican male diagnosed with cholangiocarcinoma, a cancer that begins in the bile ducts, was hospitalized with weakness and abdominal pain. He was suffering from sepsis, and his disease had progressed.

Mr. J was offered palliative chemotherapy but declined it, preferring his own remedy of "bitters and herbs." But no one wanted to address that preference.

While hospitalized, Mr. J began experiencing visions of his deceased mother, which comforted him. He had no psychotic symptoms or fluctuation of consciousness and no history of prior psychiatric disturbances or substance use problems.

As the medical team had concerns about Mr. J's mental status and treatment decisions, a psychiatric consult was requested. Psychiatry felt that Mr. J lacked capacity due to confusion, limited insight/judgment, and impaired understanding of the benefits and risks of the recommended palliative oncologic treatment. To help establish goals of care, a palliative care consult was requested.

During his meeting with the palliative care team, Mr. J reflected upon his life, expressing regret over past choices that caused divorce and estrangement from his daughter—an only child. He was aware of his cancer progression and proximity to death. He wished to make his own medical decisions, stating he did not want resuscitation or intubation in case of cardiac arrest or to be kept alive by machines. Most important to him was to go home and take his own "bitters, herbs, and cleansing regimen."

Religion and Spirituality

Mr. J also confided that he saw his mother twice, although he knew it was not logical because she was deceased. When his mother appeared, she told him he would be "joining her in her world soon." He was not frightened by the visions and expressed the comfort and peace he experienced from these encounters. Throughout the interview, Mr. J remained attentive, calm, and rational.

The palliative care team concluded that Mr. J had the capacity to make decisions about EOL care. However, the initial determination of lack of capacity remained. The patient's daughter was contacted and agreed to act as his surrogate decision-maker. Although apprised of her father's expressed wishes, Mr. J's daughter felt the burden of decision-making for a parent from whom she was estranged. Understanding him as someone who "lived life to the fullest," she opted for all life-sustaining treatments, including cardiopulmonary resuscitation. Subsequently, Mr. J suffered cardiac arrest, was resuscitated and intubated, and transferred to the intensive care unit, where he died shortly thereafter.

Exit Strategies

MEET MRS. C, A CHINESE WOMAN WITH MARKS BEHIND HER EARS

When I met her in the hospital, Mrs. C was cheerful but disappointed. In her 70s, she was gradually declining in function, and her ability to get around and do things for herself was limited. She'd been listening to Chinese radio shows and learned about advance directives and that here in America (in New York), people could make their own decisions about end-of-life care. Although she liked this approach, she never discussed her wishes with her two daughters. Mrs. C told me she would not have minded "dying in my sleep."

Then she got sicker with bad pneumonia and had to come to the hospital. Eventually her lung function deteriorated and then her heart stopped. Her daughters decided for "full code," which means proceeding with resuscitation measures, intubation (putting an airway tube down her throat and windpipe), and placing her on life support. To secure the tube in place, medical tape would be wrapped around the tube, then across her face, behind her ears, and around the back of her head. Mrs. C was sedated into a medical coma during her stay in the intensive care unit (ICU) so that she would not pull out the tube that was meant to save her life.

After about a week in the ICU, she got better. The sedation was lightened, the tape was cut, and the tube removed/pulled out from her airway. She had a sore throat for a couple of days but got better. As I spoke with Mrs. C, she was absolutely certain that she had died and almost gone to heaven but stated that her daughters and the nurses "pulled me back down."

"How do you know you almost went to heaven?" I asked.

"I feel the marks behind my ears. I was marked in heaven, but then they pulled me back down here," she explained.

"I see. How do you feel about all this?" I was very curious.

"I wish they didn't do that. I was ready. What's the point of coming back down? So I can have more time to get weaker? I'm ready."

ONE STEP CLOSER TO HEAVEN

I will always remember Percy, my patient with advanced cancer. She was staying in the hospital and couldn't wash her hair. It was getting matted up, so she decided to shave it. I thought she may have lost her hair due to chemotherapy treatments. Nope!

"I had my daughter shave it off, because nobody was going to wash my hair anyway," she said.

Wow! I asked her if she was Buddhist due to her bald head.

"No, I'm Christian," she said. She proceeded to tell me how faithful she was. She was diagnosed with cancer three years before at another hospital, and they had a whole plan for her because it was still in an early stage and surgically treatable. However, she never followed up, believing firmly that God would heal her. Now the cancer had spread and was not treatable. Percy was at the end of her life.

Even as the cancer advanced, she didn't waver in her faith. She asked me about my faith and explained her desire to convert me. This wasn't my favorite part of the conversation.

Breathe in. Breathe out.

I focused back on her care. We held a family meeting at her bedside, with Percy, me, her daughter, and the nurse.

"At this point, given that you have this very serious condition, what's important to you?" I asked.

"I want to continue to pray and to help people, hear the Lord, spread the word of Christ, and help them go to heaven and not hell," Percy said. She didn't want to talk about cancer, saying, "I don't want to focus on that; it's not important." She just wanted to keep preaching.

She had told a different team that if she wanted "full code"—if her heart stopped—she wanted to be placed on ventilators and resuscitated, which didn't make much sense, given her worsening condition and the fact that she declined all her treatments. Instead of making demands or challenging her, I burrowed deeper on what mattered most to her.

"We respect what you say, and it really seems like your faith is the most important thing," I said.

"Yes!" she responded.

"How about if we make three medical recommendations?"

"Okay."

"Number one, we're gonna get your pain and your other symptoms under control so we can give you the best quality of life, and you can pray and do the things that you love the most. How about that?"

"Yes," she said resoundingly.

"Okay. Number two, since you're really devoted to Jesus Christ and heaven, and your disease has progressed, the good news is that you're one step closer to heaven," I said. As the words came out of my mouth, I felt her daughter stiffen up next to me. I thought the nurse was going to faint.

Percy beamed with the brightest smile yet. "That's great," she said.

Religion and Spirituality

"Yes, it's great," I reaffirmed. Smiling along with her, behind my mask.

"Okay. Number three, as your disease continues to advance, at some point, your heart is going to stop and you're going to stop breathing. At that point, you're going to die. We're not going to put you on machines or anything to put distance between you and God. We're gonna let you go peacefully to heaven and unite with God."

"Yes," she said. "Okay."

"We have a paper to sign for that. Are you willing to sign it?" I asked.

"Yes," Percy said.

Before we concluded our meeting, I asked Percy to lead us in a prayer for our wellbeing and salvation. Percy happily obliged and prayed fervently for us for five minutes.

Whew. I stepped outside of her room, and her daughter followed me out.

"That was really great. We've been trying to get through to her for so long—that was wonderful. The way you put it just made sense," the daughter said.

The nurse told me later, "I can't believe you told her she was one step closer to heaven—and that she liked it."

Silently, I thought to myself. I can't believe I said that either. But words just came out of my mouth. Perhaps it was divine intervention?

Every patient is different, and my goal as they face their final chapter of life is to listen to them and tap into their greatest needs. Palliative care doctors are problem solvers, planners, concierges, and pragmatists. They are tasked with putting puzzle pieces together and giving each patient a specialized care plan—aligning treatment recommendations and plans with their wants and needs.

LESSONS

- People have cultural-, spiritual-, or faith-related interpretations and preferences when making end-of-life decisions. It's important to ask

Religion and Spirituality

about them and for us to all share our thoughts with our families and our doctors.

- Experiment using the FICA[6] approach to think about your faith, involvement, community, and how you would want your doctors and healthcare professionals to address your faith concerns.
- Miracles sometimes do happen, so don't lose hope! Share your "miracle" scenario with your care team. Keep wishing for a miracle while also making other plans just in case.
- It's always good to hope for "Plan A," and have a "Plan B" as back up! I heard a presentation from Marilu Henner once, and she really advocates for having a Plan B!

---

6   Tami Borneman, Betty Ferrell, and Christina M. Puchalski, "Evaluation of the FICA Tool for Spiritual Assessment," *Journal of Pain and Symptom Management* 40, no. 2 (2010): 163–173, https://doi.org/10.1016/j.jpainsymman.2009.12.019.

CHAPTER 10

Birthdays

BIRTHDAYS ARE SUPER IMPORTANT! IN SOME ways, I think we have birthday celebrations backward. In many cultures, there are big celebrations when a baby turns one year old—elaborate blue or pink cakes, streamers and decorations, gifts and presents, and sometimes even firecrackers.

That's even though the baby is too young to even remember the party!

As we age, the parties typically get less and less elaborate. Some adults don't make a big deal of it, while others go all-out for the five- and 10-year milestones. When I turned 50, my husband organized a huge surprise party. I had no idea—I thought he forgot about it. He even got help from my kids, family, and friends to pull the wool over my eyes. It was a wonderful, amazing, truly memorable party!

Just because someone is facing the end of their life doesn't mean their birthday isn't worth celebrating. Instead, it represents even more reason to go all-out.

I want to share stories of two patients who experienced special birthdays during the final chapters of their lives.

RECONNECTING WITH A LOVED ONE

Mr. Jones was a patient of mine who received hospice care at home. He was almost 90 years old and had advanced heart failure. He wanted to stay home for his final days and not be moved to a nursing home. He was divorced and had no children. He was at odds with his only little brother, Jack, and they had not spoken for years. Mr. Jones overcame his fear and told the hospice chaplain about his dying wish—to make it to his 90th birthday and have a "big birthday bash," to which he could invite all his friends to come reminisce old times together and say goodbye. Most importantly, he wanted to use this opportunity to reach out to Jack! Once Mr. Jones expressed this goal, his hospice team jolted to action. The chaplain and the aide got to work. The chaplain was excellent at coordinating events and helped Mr. Jones make a list, plan out the food, the date and time, and design the invitation. The aide was very hands-on, too. She helped Mr. Jones write out the invitations and took them to the post office to send them out. Both supported Mr. Jones and gave him the courage to call Jack, who actually answered the phone. Jack told him that he would attend his final big bash.

On the day of the party, it was a fine Saturday, with sunshine and warmth in New York. A small group of Mr. Jones's friends attended, and he was pleasantly surprised to learn how many were still "alive and kicking." A few of them came with their own aides or family members. They shared stories from old times, laughed, drank, and ate soft textured snacks.

Then Jack showed up.

It was a truly emotional moment since Mr. Jones and Jack had not seen or talked to each other for years. They couldn't even remember why or what happened that led to the rift. Jack told Mr. Jones about his life, what he'd been up to, and that his marriage was on the rocks. As a matter of fact, Jack was thinking about divorcing his wife. Mr. Jones listened, then shared his own divorce story, the regrets he had experienced over the years, and the things that he might have done differently looking back. Jack also listened intently, and thanked Mr. Jones for his thoughts.

A few days after the party, Jack called Mr. Jones to thank him, and he wanted to try and repair his marriage based on Mr. Jones's advice. Mr. Jones told the hospice team how grateful he was for their help in making his last birthday wish come true, which included reuniting him with Jack. Now he had no regrets. He felt that even at the end of his life, he was able to give his little brother Jack a final gift. A few weeks later, Mr. Jones passed away peacefully.

MRS. A: I'M GOING HOME FOR MY THANKSGIVING BIRTHDAY!

Mrs. A was a fierce Latin woman I met in the hospital. She was in her 60s and clearly the matriarch in her family. Whatever she said, went.

Birthdays

She was admitted because she had difficulty breathing. At first she really didn't want to come to the hospital, but when her symptoms became intolerable, she came through the ER. Everyone thought she had COVID, but her tests kept coming back negative. She was usually healthy, with a touch of high blood pressure, and was still working. She was in the hospital for three weeks and received one test after another. A small effusion building up in her lung was found, but she was negative for COVID-19. She was using maximum oxygen and other measures, though her oxygen numbers were still low. Oxygen levels needed to increase before she could be medically released.

From early on, Mrs. A made it known to all her doctors and nurses that she did *not* want to be intubated and live on artificial breathing machines.

I met Mrs. A when I was called in to provide a palliative care consult. It was a difficult situation where Mrs. A was not improving after weeks of treatment, she did not want to be intubated, and she was now insisting on going home, but her oxygen levels were still low and not safe to meet medical discharge standards.

Exit Strategies

When I first met Mrs. A, she was distant and aloof and did not want to talk to me. She was tired of being in the hospital and not getting any answers. She felt like a caged animal and didn't know where to turn. She did give me permission to speak with her daughter Nikki, who meant the world to her, but they could hardly see each other because of limited visitation hours during the COVID pandemic. I tried my best to facilitate Nikki being allowed in to visit Mrs. A and stay a bit longer during visits.

After another few days, we decided to hold a family meeting with Mrs. A, Nikki, the medical team, and the palliative care team. I served as the meeting facilitator. We came to understand that Mrs. A felt that she was in limbo and wasn't getting better. She knew she might get worse, and if she did, she would not want invasive procedures or be intubated on machines. She was ready to go home and try her luck. She said she was a God-loving woman and had faith no matter what happened. Nikki was willing to support her.

The hospitalist (the doctor guiding her treatment at the hospital) was concerned about what would happen if Mrs. A went home. He was worried that she wouldn't survive very long, and that the hospital could wind up getting sued for providing poor medical care.

I suggested that we try a "wean down" of her oxygen and see how she responded. If she felt okay, even with reduced oxygen levels and oxygen saturation numbers, perhaps she could go home.

Mrs. A and Nikki were very interested in trying this out and saw a ray of hope for going home. Nikki called me later that day to say that Thanksgiving was coming, and it also happened to be Mrs. A's birthday. Mrs. A was determined to go home for her Thanksgiving birthday!

We tried the weaning down oxygen in the next 24 hours. Mrs. A actually felt okay. And even though her oxygen saturation numbers were lower than we preferred, she was awake, alert, responsive, talkative, and adamant that she wished to go home.

We discussed that in her situation, the best solution would be to send her home on hospice care with the explicit understanding that she could die. With that being said, she would die at home, where she wanted to be. Oxygen, home care equipment, and medications would be provided to her for her comfort and to alleviate symptoms.

"That's what I want," she said. "In two days it will be Thanksgiving and my birthday. I need to leave tomorrow."

It was still a difficult thing for the medical team and hospitalist doctor to accept. But what was the alternative? Keep Mrs. A in the hospital for another four weeks? Did she have four more weeks? What were we going to provide for her that we hadn't already tried? Can we keep people against their will? Mrs. A was of sound mind, understood the risks, and repeatedly expressed her wish to go home. If she was going to die, she wanted to die at home.

Finally, everyone agreed. We worked together with our case managers and sent Mrs. A home late on the Wednesday before Thanksgiving. Seeing her smile was priceless. After she left, I was afraid to call them to check on what happened. But on Friday afternoon, I got up the courage to call Nikki. To my surprise, Nikki was upbeat and happy.

Birthdays

"My mom is doing great. She's so happy to be home! We had a wonderful Thanksgiving and she had her favorite cake for her birthday. There's *no place* like home. Thank you!" she said.

LESSONS

- If you feel like having a birthday party, or any party, have it! What a great reason to celebrate!
- Just because someone is facing the end of their life doesn't mean their birthday isn't worth celebrating. Instead, it represents even more reason to go all-out.
- There's no place like home!

CHAPTER 11

Using the Right Words

SO MUCH OF OUR MEDICAL TERMINOLOGY IS about success and failure, winning and losing.

Someone *failed* an assessment or chemotherapy.

They *lost* their battle with cancer.

We should get away from using those words. School is pass-fail, sure, but a patient didn't fail their speech and swallow tests. Instead, the speech and swallow testing revealed that the patient was at high risk for aspiration.

Patients are going through enough already. They don't need to face the stigma of "failure" on top of that. A patient didn't fail with their chemotherapy treatments—the chemo treatments didn't stop the spread of the cancer. And doctors feel bad enough, too. But the doctors also did not "fail"—they tried their best to help, and the treatment did not work in this case.

Another loaded phrase is "pulling the plug." I don't like that term. It sounds cruel, as though you are actively doing something to end the person's life. The actual term, palliative extubation, simply means we are no longer intervening. It's freeing the body of artificial assistance and allowing the body to do what it does. Another way to think about it is "compassionate liberation from ventilator support."

Palliative extubations[7]—which are covered in the next chapter—are difficult and complex, and they represent one of the hardest decisions a relative or patient can make. As you face these circumstances, I want you to have the right vocabulary. We need to be a little more objective and less judgmental regarding the words we use.

---

7   Christina Ortega-Chen et al., "Palliative Extubation: A Discussion of Practices and Considerations," *Journal of Pain and Symptom Management*, 66, no. 2 (2023): 219–231, https://doi.org/10.1016/j.jpainsymman.2023.03.011.

Using the Right Words

LESSONS

- We should get away from using loaded words such as winning or losing, passing or failing, when describing someone's medical status.
- Patients are going through enough already! They don't need to face the stigma of failure on top of that. Let's think carefully about the words we use.
- Be mindful about the words you use! Try to approach someone with a compassionate mindset, not a blaming or judging mindset.

CHAPTER 12

Palliative Extubation: Disconnecting from the Ventilator

Nowadays, medicine has many interventions that can artificially prolong the living process. One of the most common is a mechanical ventilator, which can keep patients alive who have acute respiratory failure.

People who are intubated have a tube stuck from their mouth into their trachea (or air pipe). Then they're connected to the ventilator, or respirator, to artificially breathe for them.

For those who are unfamiliar with ventilators, it can be jarring to encounter them. One time, I brought my son to the hospital to pick up something from my office. While walking by a medical unit, my son was struck by a cacophony of humming and beeping sounds.

"What's that sound, mom?"

"That's the ventilator. It's a form of artificial life support machine that breathes for patients who cannot breathe on their own."

"It sounds like Darth Vader."

THE TRUTH ABOUT LIVING ON A VENTILATOR

The hope is always that the patient can get better, get off the ventilator, and go back to their normal function. But sometimes that doesn't materialize.

The next option is living permanently on the ventilator, which requires a tracheostomy—a hole being cut on the front of the neck so a tube can be inserted. Most patients in this situation also can't swallow naturally, so an artificial feeding tube is surgically placed in their stomach, and the patients are fed through the tube.

Many patients living on a ventilator are not conscious. Some are awake but not aware of what their

Palliative Extubation: Disconnecting from the Ventilator

medical condition is and lack capacity to make their own medical decisions. They often travel back and forth from the hospital to the nursing home due to infections that are hard to prevent once the patients are immunocompromised, with artificial holes in their bodies that become portals for bacteria. When caring for patients like this, I feel like I'm in the movie *Coma*, rounding and walking by people who are in suspended animation.

As one nurse described it to me, "These patients are dying inch by inch." Often, because these patients cannot even turn themselves in bed, they remain in one position for a prolonged period of time, and they develop pressure ulcers or "bed sores," which become a portal of infection, a source of pain, and a sign of deterioration. But family members may not see the bed sores, because healthcare professionals try their best to keep the patients cleaned up and nicely covered when families visit.

Palliative extubation—the removal of a patient's ventilator—is an option available to patients and their families, but one that requires medical, ethical, and moral considerations.

KNOWING WHAT TO ASK YOUR DOCTOR

These scenarios aren't easy to consider—and that's exactly why I want you to start thinking about them. It's okay to think about the hard things in advance.

When doctors ask you questions like "What do you want us to do? Do you want us to do everything?" They mean putting a tube down your throat and connecting you to the ventilator, hoping for the best, and not necessarily thinking about whether or not you would come out of it.

When faced with these choices, it's important to ask questions so you can gather the information you need to make the right decision for you. These include:

- "What are my chances of getting better and getting off the ventilator? Be honest with me."
- "What are my other options?"
- "Can I speak with the palliative care team to get more information?"

It is also critically important to tell the doctors and medical teams about who you are, what truly matters to you, and what an acceptable quality of life means to you. For some people, quantity of life is more important than quality: as long as they have a breath left, even if they are in a coma, it is good enough. For others, quality of life reigns: they want to be awake, recognize their families, be independent and take care of themselves, not burden others, and be able to travel or move around.

Just because a medical intervention is being offered does not mean that it's recommended. It may just be a last resort or last-ditch effort—something to do to avoid telling you bad news.

THANKFULLY, WE HAVE OPTIONS

If you or a loved one does end up intubated on the ventilator, it's important to know that you have options. Fortunately, we live in a country where U.S. laws support patient-centered care and shared decision-making between patients and medical professionals.

The Patient Self Determination Act of 1990[8] allows patients to drive their own medical decisions.

---

8   Dac Teoli and Sassan Ghassamzadah, "Patient Self-Determination Act," Treasure

Ventilators, antibiotics, and feeding tubes are all medical interventions. Just because those interventions are available doesn't mean a patient needs to receive them or that they need to keep using them once they've been provided.

You have the option to withdraw or stop medical interventions that are not working for you or serving your goals. I have witnessed hundreds of patients and their families make the difficult decision to withdraw from the ventilator and allow a natural passing, known as "palliative extubation."

This is a decision not made lightly! There should be family meetings and discussions about the pros and cons, the process, and what to expect.

STEP BY STEP

The conversations leading up to palliative extubation go step by step. When we meet with families of patients who have serious illnesses, we always want to

---

Island, StatPearls Publishing, last modified August 28, 2023, https://www.ncbi.nlm.nih.gov/books/NBK538297/.

start by asking them what they've been told by doctors up to this point.

They should have some reasonable understanding of the serious nature or the end-state nature of things because you can't really make decisions if you don't know the patient's medical situation and prognosis.

Once they have a realistic understanding of the prognosis, then we can explore further and learn what's important to them, what matters in their life, and their values.

HIGHER POWER

Everyone wants to know how long a patient will survive following palliative extubation—and we often tell families, "Now it's up to a higher power."

At that point, it's not up to us anymore. There are certain indicators that the process could be shorter or longer depending on blood pressure or mental status, but at the end, it's up to a higher power. If you believe in God, it's up to God. If you believe in something else, it's up to something else.

It's not up to us.

Having said that, I do ask my patients and families to be emotionally prepared for a wide range of time. Based on my research, after being disconnected from the ventilator, life expectancy could be minutes, hours, or days. Families, as well as medical teams, may get nervous if the patient lingers for days. However, when you really examine the situation, the big picture has not changed. The timeframe for the dying process can vary, just like the birthing process.

ADDITIONAL RESOURCES

Often, before palliative extubation, it's a good idea to enroll the patient in hospice care for extra support, symptom management, and bereavement support. Patients who are undergoing palliative extubation are at the end of life. The expectation is that they will likely pass away soon after, but the timeframe can vary. The patient may also have symptoms including breathing distress, pain, secretions, anxiety, and agitation. Family members may not know what to expect or where to turn for support. Enrolling the patient in hospice care can provide extra support for the patient *and* the family. The hospice team can work with the hospital team to better monitor symptoms, titrate (or change medications to control symptoms), and answer family's questions. Once the patient dies, hospice organizations provide bereavement or grief support for family members who need these services. These are built-in services mandated by Medicare and can be quite helpful.

MOM, OPEN YOUR EYES

Some people struggle with making the decision to remove a loved one's ventilator—they're painstaking about it and have to go over every single detail. Others are very clear, sure, and direct.

I had a Latin American patient with severe lung disease. The patient had been intubated four times already—every time she got off the ventilator, she was soon intubated again. In this instance it was unlikely that she would come off the ventilator. Her lung function was failing.

While intubated, she kept her eyes closed and didn't talk to anybody, which made us believe that she didn't have capacity. So we spoke to her daughter about the situation and discussed the options of doing a tracheostomy or taking her off the ventilator. Either way, she was going to pass away soon. She was at the end stage of her life.

Her daughter just couldn't make that decision. She brought in her husband and he deferred, as he was the son-in-law. He said, "I am just here to support my wife."

"Smart man," I thought.

After a few days of the daughter struggling to decide, the nurse let us know that the patient had been opening her eyes—and she believed the patient might have the capacity to respond to requests.

So we went to talk to her and brought her daughter in the room.

Palliative Extubation: Disconnecting from the Ventilator

"Mom, open your eyes," she said, and the patient opened her eyes.

"You've been on the ventilator for a few days now, and we have some serious things we have to discuss with you," I told her. "Your lungs, they're bad. You've been on this four times before, and the situation isn't improving, so we have to make a decision. We can make a hole in your throat, and you'd be connected to a ventilator, and you could live like that." At that, she shook her head "no."

I continued. "Alternatively, we could take it out. But you could die."

She shook her head up and down, "yes."

Her daughter was so relieved. "Thank God, it's a Christmas miracle. My mother's making her own decisions."

These were big decisions, and I wanted to give the patient a chance to think about it overnight and ask her the same questions again. I wrote the whole thing down and asked her the set of questions the next day, and the patient chose palliative extubation. At that point, I discussed the next steps with the daughter.

"You have to be emotionally prepared, because it could be minutes or hours, but she will stop breathing," I said.

We pre-medicated the patient before taking her off the ventilator so she was comfortable and not struggling. The goal was to keep the patient comfortable and peaceful.

It was Christmas Eve, and as we anticipated, the patient stopped breathing. I got a call from the staff on the unit—they had to call rapid response on the daughter because she threw herself on the ground.

"Should we re-intubate the patient?" they asked me.

"No," I said. "The patient doesn't want it anymore, and the daughter said that she accepted her mother making her own decisions." They wound up taking the daughter to the Emergency Department.

It's very hard when our relatives die. But in a case like this, the patient made her own decision across multiple conversations, and the patient was consistent in her wishes.

Palliative Extubation: Disconnecting from the Ventilator

GETTING EVERYONE ON THE SAME PAGE

It's so important to get the person's wishes and perspectives—and the situations where patients were able to decide on palliative extubation, while rare, have been so impactful for me.

Joe was my patient who had ALS, or Lou Gehrig's Disease. The disease robbed him of muscle function even while his mind remained sharp. He started to lose strength from the bottom up. He lost the ability to walk or move, then he couldn't use his hands and arms, and eventually he couldn't use his respiratory muscles—at which point he was intubated. When he couldn't swallow, he needed a feeding tube, and in the meantime, he experienced and felt everything.

He was frozen in his body but he still had mental capacity.

Joe ended up in a nursing home with a ventilator and a feeding tube. He came back time after time with sepsis and infections. The first time I met with Joe, I liked him right away. Even though he couldn't talk or make sounds, he had beautiful, expressive eyes that gave you answers. Eyes that could pierce through your soul. He could mouth words and somehow made it easy for me to read his lips. After we got to know each better, I talked to him about his care options, including palliative extubation.

"Coming off the ventilator is an option," I told him.

"No, I think I'm gonna stay on," he said.

"I just want you to know, because people's wishes change, and the quality-of-life changes."

Joe was sent to a nursing home and came back not long after, and at that point, he said, "I started this conversation with my family." He didn't want his family members to judge him or feel like he was giving up. His family was pushing back on his wishes, and he wanted to have a family meeting.

So we gathered his sons and other family members and had a conversation about his life.

"My quality of life is getting worse and worse," Joe told them. "I'm staring at the ceiling every day in a

Palliative Extubation: Disconnecting from the Ventilator

nursing home, not able to do anything, and I don't want that."

There were a lot of tears. But at that point, there wasn't a decision to be made—it was just a chance to talk and get everyone's feelings out. The patient was treated for his infection and went back to the nursing home.

When Joe came back a third time, his family called us.

"We think that he's ready," they told us.

So we had another family meeting to confirm. They'd all had a chance to think things over, and they were supportive of his decision. They weren't judging him. They'd seen how he was suffering and didn't want him to suffer anymore.

The day of the palliative extubation, his whole family came. The chaplain was also there, and there were lots of prayers as we prepared the patient. We knew that he wouldn't live long after the palliative extubation—the disease had taken away his respiratory function and muscles.

We were all standing there, the prayers had been said, and everyone was around the bed waiting for me to give the order to proceed with medication. This was followed by the removal of the ventilator.

Joe stared at me with his piercing eyes.

"Are you ready?" he asked me, mouthing the words. "Because I'm ready when you're ready."

I had been through this process many times before, and yet, the emotions in this case were so overwhelming because everything would happen so quickly. *I'm not ready,* I thought.

Four minutes.

After we removed the ventilator, the patient was free of his awful, horrible disease in four minutes. He had been trapped, and his whole family was very grateful that there was a way out for him.

Two days later, I received a beautiful gift basket from his family to thank me for freeing Joe's soul.

Palliative Extubation: Disconnecting from the Ventilator

LESSONS

- It's important to understand what palliative extubation entails.
- Patients in the U.S. have options—something that shouldn't be taken for granted. Patients and their families should ask about those options and choose those that are the best match for them. You may not always be told about every option if you don't ask about them.
- There can be religious, ethical, and moral factors at play when considering palliative extubation, so be sure it's something that is acceptable to you and your community. You can also ask the hospital's ethics committee to speak with you or answer questions you may have.

CHAPTER 13

Facing My Mortality During My COVID Illness

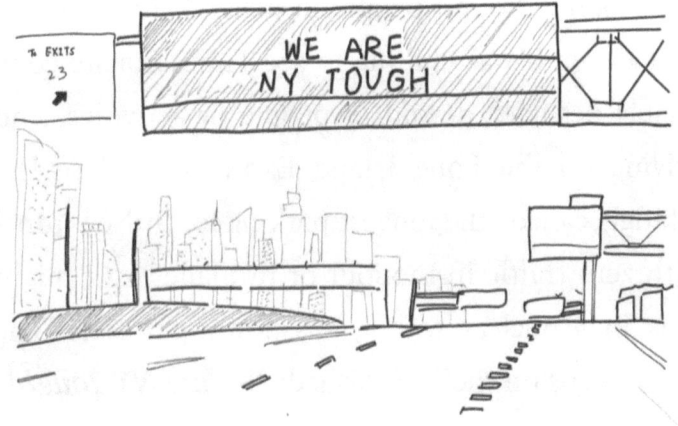

As a palliative care physician, I regularly encounter illness, functional decline, and death through the daily encounters with my patients. But the COVID-19 pandemic in March of 2020 gave me new insight into the uncertainty and fear that often surrounds end-of-life care.

Exit Strategies

The COVID-19 pandemic hit New York like a storm—in a matter of weeks, the city became the pandemic's epicenter. People of all ages were getting sick. Those that struggled to breathe would go to the hospital. Far too many didn't improve, and within days, they were dead.

We tried to socially distance and wear masks and avoid being around people in general. The city was shut down. It was chilling to see Times Square completely desolate, devoid of people or activities. And driving on the Long Island Expressway (the LIE), jokingly called "the longest parking lot in New York," with zero traffic in the four or five lanes as it might look in a nuclear winter, was downright eerie. The traffic signs on the LIE flashed: *"We are NY Tough!"*

It was a horrifying time. And on March 26, 2020, I became one of New York City's 3,101 new cases of COVID-19.[9] On that fateful Thursday, I went to work despite a mild cough—allergies, I thought.

---

9   Jonah Engel Bromwich, et al., "N.Y.C. Death Toll Hits 365 as Case Tops 23,000," New York Times, last modified March 27, 2020, https://www.nytimes.com/2020/03/26/nyregion/coronavirus-new-york-update.html.

But it wasn't allergies.

By noon, chills and severe muscle aches possessed my body. I was sluggish and tired. I could not even get up from my office chair.

As a healthcare professional with symptoms, I was able to get COVID-tested that afternoon. I drove to the testing site for the nasal swab. I parked in the parking lot as instructed and a doctor fully geared with personal protective equipment came to do my swab. When she reached my car window, she said, "Dr. Pan!" It was a medicine resident whom I knew.

I said, "Thank you, and please be safe."

After the swab, I felt more chills and even weaker. I mustered up my remaining energy and concentration and made the drive home. I parked the car and went into my house. I announced to my husband and boys, "I think I have COVID. I have to quarantine myself in my room. I have zero energy left." I went to my bed and fell asleep.

WORRIED SICK

The next few days were a blur. I received a call the following day from my primary care colleague. "I have bad news. You are COVID positive," she said. My husband and kids made me soup and hot tea, leaving them outside my bedroom door. I would pick it up and eat or drink whatever I could. Sleep. Go to the restroom. Sleep. The next time I truly awoke, it was Monday.

Monday. I felt reasonably rested. *Maybe the worst is over,* I thought. *Maybe I'll be able to make a fast recovery.* I hoped to be able to return to work soon.

Then the COVID storm restarted. Severe cluster headaches, cough, fever, more chills, and profound fatigue. I could imagine the virus traveling throughout my body. I tried to but could not take deep breaths because it would cause a coughing spiral, leading to a headache that was so severe that all I could do was hold my head and moan or cry.

My mother was worried sick. She and my brother brought me homemade soup and other good Chinese food. I have always been active on social media and

Facing My Mortality During My COVID Illness

I posted that I was sick with COVID-19. I received tremendous support from my family and friends from all walks of my life: high school, college, medical school, work friends, and colleagues from past and present. Friends and relatives would call me but I was too weak to answer. I was grateful to have this kind of support while I was in quarantine! I also received sound advice, including:

- "Listen to your body. Get the rest you need. Don't rush it."
- "Try sleeping in different positions. Try proning and avoid lying on your back—it helps with oxygenation."
- "Guilt is an ugly feeling. We need to get it out of our systems. Being responsible and respectful of ourselves is something we all deserve."

BRAIN FOG

For the next week or so, I became best friends with W.A.T.O. (water, acetaminophen, thermometer, and oximeter). I started taking acetaminophen because of my high fevers and headaches. I remember calculating how much acetaminophen I needed to take to get pain and fever relief, yet not impair my liver function. I tracked the time to see if I could make it for five or six hours so that I could take the next dose. I began journaling my temperatures and medication dosing.

Another scary symptom that I experienced is what I called my COVID brain (now it's called COVID brain fog). For the first few days, I could not think clearly and my judgment was impaired. Some colleagues called me to discuss initiatives, not knowing that I was out sick. I tried my best to give input. Retrospectively, I was giving unclear suggestions and making bad decisions. After a while, I told my colleagues that I was out sick and not in any position to make important decisions.

Some nights, facing delirium and disorientation, I wasn't sure if I was the patient or the doctor. For example, I would cough and get short of breath and tell myself, "This is the time to sleep prone." I would get into a prone position, and think, "Good, this is good for the patient." Then I would say to myself,

"Snap out of it—*you* are the patient. Just focus on yourself right now."

I later read an article about COVID-19 having neurological impacts on patients and found myself recognizing many of the experiences I faced.

LOW POINTS AND STRONG OPINIONS

I had splitting headaches and started to get short of breath. I checked my own oxygen saturation and it kept going down, down, down.

Because of my ongoing cough, especially at night, I could not sleep and get proper rest.

Some nights, at my lowest points, I worried that I wasn't going to make it. I wasn't ready to leave my husband and kids behind.

But I also had strong opinions about my care. After seeing what happened with some of the patients brought into the hospital and how a lot of them didn't go home, I told my husband that I didn't want to go to the hospital nor be on a ventilator—I preferred having oxygen at home and taking my chances.

He supported my wishes, but he didn't agree.

"If I got COVID, I want to go to the nearest hospital that has a trial for Remdesivir," he said. "Put me on a machine, do whatever you can, and then we'll talk."

Wow, I thought. Even though we were married all of these years—and both had medical backgrounds—our wishes for care were completely different. This situation helped me to understand why so many people facing end-of-life care prefer to receive care at home.

HOW DO YOU NOT KNOW?

As I faced the worst of my COVID crisis, my energy was completely sapped—I couldn't even get up.

My husband got me some potato chips, and I guess I had a strange taste side effect with my COVID, because those chips tasted a million times saltier than normal, as though I were drinking ocean water, or just pouring a salt shaker over my tongue.

It all made me think about my patients when their bodies breaking down. How they must feel isolated from the people they love—how terrible it is when nothing tastes or feels normal.

I didn't know what was happening to me—just as my patients often don't know what's happening to them, either. They're forced to answer questions all the time about how they feel, and when they say they don't know, you think, *how do you not know?* But here I was, with all of my medical experience, and I genuinely didn't know, either.

A NEW OUTLOOK

I thought a lot about my patients as I lay, alone, wondering if I was going to survive. That experience has stuck with me for a long time. I've always tried to do my best to put myself in the patient's shoes and understand their needs, but I've never been directly in that spot myself before. Going through that ordeal made me even more patient-focused, and more patient, too.

I've also found myself embracing my emotions. I remember the day I returned to work after so much time away. I arrived at the hospital, parked my car, and walked up to the front entrance. As I looked up at the name of my hospital and our community's supportive messages taped in the windows, I couldn't help but cry. One message in particular stuck with me: *"We are NY Tough."*

Before COVID, if I had a choice between laughing something off or crying about it, I would always choose laughter. After COVID, I gained the freedom to cry whenever I feel like it—and that's okay! Crying was therapeutic and liberating, and it helped me vent my emotions instead of hiding or suppressing them. I realized that life is too short to suppress my emotions.

LESSONS

- Experiencing sickness or illness can be horrible. But it can also give you a window of compassion for others. In my case, being sick with COVID helped me to better understand and

empathize with my patients who told me they were out of breath.
- Life is fragile. Remember to appreciate the little things in life: the rose petals, the fresh crisp air, the smell of freshly made coffee, the steam from good soup, and the hug from your child.
- Keep an attitude of gratitude. Be grateful for the people in your life!
- Here your chance to write the names of three people you appreciate:

_____

_____

_____

- Try writing three NEW things you are grateful for:

_____

_____

CHAPTER 14

Find an Excuse to Celebrate or Make a Bucket List

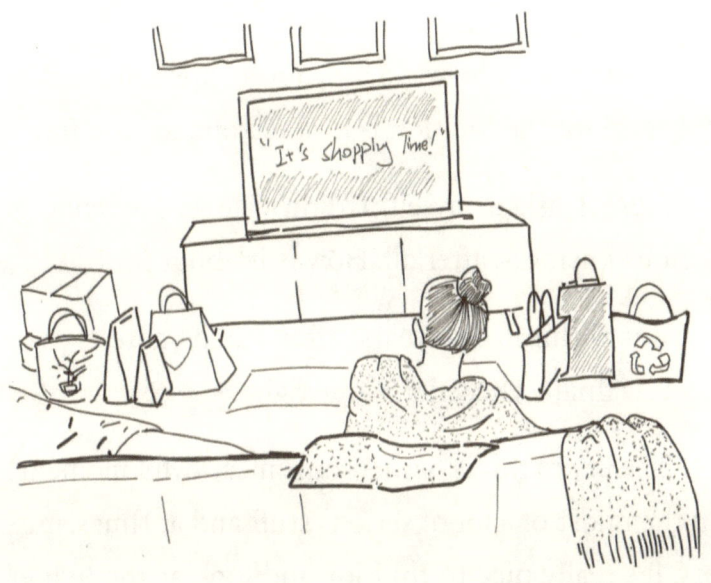

It's easy to take things too seriously, espe-cially when it involves palliative care. But we shouldn't forget about fun.

Exit Strategies

I remember when I first became an attending physician after finishing my training. I didn't have a lot of experience. We were doing our attending rounds and normally went around and introduced ourselves before we talked about our goals for the rotation. Some were saying things like, "I want to learn about electrolyte disorders," or explained their interest in other topics.

An attendee who was a little more experienced said, "My goal for the rotation is for everyone to have fun."

Huh? I asked myself. I didn't agree. Medicine is serious business, after all. How is it about fun?

But within a few years, after I had more experience, it finally clicked. He was right.

The key to this is having some nice, joyful moments in the midst of a lot of serious stuff and at times, misery. It's really nice to find joy and look at the lighter side of things. Life is short, you know?

I've since become known for celebrations. My boss will say, "Cynthia's having one of her celebrations again. Must be somebody's birthday, or maybe nothing at all."

Find an Excuse to Celebrate or Make a Bucket List

Somebody did a nice presentation? Celebration time.

Somebody passes the board exam? Celebration time.

A nice letter from a patient? Celebration time.

Too often, in life and in work, people only get called out when something goes wrong. Why not call someone out for doing something right and give positive feedback?

The people around me now keep track of birthdays for our team members, and they're in charge of bringing cake—I don't even need to worry about it.

That festive approach applies to patients too, and we celebrate them and try to honor their wishes every chance we get.

ANNA'S LOVE FOR QVC

Whenever I visited Anna at home, she was always laying comfortably on her sofa, cuddled up in her various colorful throws and watching QVC. Whether I was there for a routine visit or to drain fluid from her abdominal catheter, the channel was always on. The hostess and models would be talking about earrings, shoes, blouses, and the fantastic features they would all have.

These brought back memories for me, because when I was training as a medicine resident doctor I would always binge watch QVC. I was able to acquire some fun jewelry as a result.

Since Anna and I both shared a love for "retail therapy," these were nice visits for both of us. I would set up the draining system and hook it up to the catheter in her abdomen, then sit down and chat. If her symptoms were under good control and she was comfortable, Anna and I would just sit and watch QVC together.

It just happened that day QVC was showing a Sherpa throw! It looked velvety soft, luxurious, and cozy. Anna was very interested in it because she was always cold after losing weight from having cancer. I asked Anna if she really needed another throw since I could see she has several already in her living room.

"It's one of my last pleasures. I can't go out and shop because I'm too weak. But thanks to QVC, I can shop all I want at home! Besides, I worked so hard all my life and saved up quite a bit of money. I am not married and don't have kids. Who am I saving the money for? Might as well spend it on myself and help out QVC!"

I nodded in agreement. She was not wrong.

"Also, I am responsible and have the money to pay for stuff I buy. But let's say I run out of money, so what? Are they going to come after me in my grave?"

We smiled at each other and turned our attention back to QVC. Now they were showing some beautiful Diamonique hoop earrings! I was feeling quite tempted and made a mental note that when I got home that night: I should go on QVC and check out those earrings!

It was time to take out the catheter. The ascites fluid ceased to come out, and the large bottle was filled with straw-colored fluid. Anna tolerated the drainage just fine with no pain. We had a great time watching QVC, which was Anna's way of optimizing her quality of life.

I packed up my equipment and said goodbye. Walking outside and taking a deep breath of the fresh air, I said a silent prayer for Anna. I felt so grateful for being able to walk, to go outside, and do the work I do.

THE LAST BROADWAY SHOW

Bernard lived somewhere on the south shore of Long Island, but he always enjoyed going into *the city* to take advantage of the cultural offerings. After he was diagnosed with pulmonary fibrosis and his symptoms kept worsening, it was harder and harder for him to go into Manhattan.

He was referred to home hospice and I went to visit him for symptom management. He was quite short of breath and was having generalized pain as well.

From the first time I met him and his family, he made it clear to me that he was not afraid of dying. He was full of life and determined to live life to the last drop. It was a breath of fresh air to speak with Bernard because he was so upbeat and hopeful no matter what the circumstance was.

Find an Excuse to Celebrate or Make a Bucket List

"Doc, just get my pain and breathing under control so I can go to Broadway and see my last show!" Bernard was a huge fan of Broadway and had seen some wonderful shows, including *A Catered Affair, Cats, A Man For All Seasons, A Tale of Two Cities, Chicago,* and *Brighton Beach Memoirs.*

His last wish was to see *The Phantom of the Opera* before he died!

One thing about working in home hospice is how rewarding it is for me as a doctor to be able to get to know my patients and what really, truly, matters to them. Also with our medical assessments, medications, and treatments, we can get our patients' symptoms under excellent control most of the time so that they can go on and accomplish their last wish(es). It's also very exciting when my patients have specific goals and wishes that we can support, and our hospice team can get behind them. In Bernard's case, it was fantastic that despite his terminal illness, he still had his mind and mental capacity to talk with us meaningfully. And yes, Bernard got to see *Phantom* and fulfilled his last wish!

Exit Strategies

SEVERAL MORE TRIPS TO SEE FAMILIES AND FRIENDS

One day out of the blue, I got a call from my nephrologist (kidney doctor) friend Nate from Oregon. He was a nephrology fellow who I trained and gave lectures and presentations to. Nate called me to thank me for teaching him serious illness communication skills, because now he's able to use them with his patients. He sees many patients who have kidney failure and receive dialysis. Dialysis usually is an ongoing treatment that takes place three times per week, with each session lasting about four to six hours. For younger and healthier patients, dialysis can be a godsend and give them a second lease on life by allowing them to continue working and making a living to support their families. For older and sicker patients, dialysis may or may not prolong their lives, can make them very fatigued, and may decrease their ability to care for themselves.

Nate was treating an elderly gentleman who had been on dialysis for a couple of years, but his condition was declining anyway. Nate had a feeling that his patient had a poor prognosis and was not going

Find an Excuse to Celebrate or Make a Bucket List

to live much longer. During one of the dialysis visits, Nate sat down with the patient and his wife and had a heart-to-heart conversation. They discussed the patient's condition, treatment course and treatment plan, and future outlook. Nate was able to hold this bad news conversation and manage the emotions around it because of the training he received when he was at my hospital. His patient and wife were grateful for Nate's honesty, caring, and commitment to take this final journey with them.

His patient decided that since time is short and while he was still able to travel, he and his wife were going to take as many trips as possible to visit their families and friends who lived scattered around the U.S.

When you take a trip knowing this is your last trip, you see it through a different lens. You appreciate every little moment and detail. You don't sweat the small stuff, and even though it was quite emotional, it was also very uplifting. Because Nate was upfront and honest with the information, his patient and wife felt empowered to be upfront and honest with their families and friends. As a result, the trip was punctuated by love, support, crying, laughing, and stories about the good old days. There were no fights, no conflicts, and none of the petty stuff that's common to occur in families.

A few weeks after they returned home the patient died. Nate received a huge gift basket from the wife to thank him for the advance notice, and for giving them the chance to have some truly special times before he died. His death was not a surprise—they had time to prepare. It was still sad, but they had no regrets. The gift basket was full of goodies that their office and dialysis unit, including patients, enjoyed.

LESSONS

- Find any reason to celebrate! Even at the end of life, you can still contribute and help someone.
- Some people are purposeful and set specific goals they wish to accomplish before their time is up. Sort of a "bucket list."
- It's a good idea to tell your doctors and healthcare team if you have specific goals and ask for their help in achieving those goals.

CHAPTER 15

People Who Plan Their Own Funerals

NOT MANY PEOPLE PLAN THEIR OWN FUNERals—and those who do are courageous!

I don't mean simply buying cemetery plots or prepaying for their funerals—I mean those who *really* thought about this seriously, took things into their own hands, and mapped out the type of ceremony they'd like to have—down to the music and structure and participants.

Planning a funeral forces you to face your own morality, which can be difficult and scary. It's easy, when thinking about your own death, to feel overwhelmed or sad or scared. It takes a very special person to go to the effort to plan out their funeral, viewing or homegoing service.

If someone is taking those steps, I like to ask them how they decided on their plans and encourage them to have fun with it—because this is kind of their last hurrah. The final celebration honoring their life.

Those who plan their own funerals tend to be planner types. Maybe they worked as event planners or are pragmatic like engineers.

It's interesting to learn what people have in mind and how they make their funeral unique or special. Maybe they use symbolic colors. One patient was focused on leaving the attendees at their funeral with a saying: "Live the life you love and love the life you live." There was another patient who made a list of her favorite books and printed it on the back of her funeral card to give to friends and family.

STAYING GRATEFUL

I once ran into a fellow doctor and was talking to her about a patient. The patient's prognosis wasn't great, and I said, "Do you ever think about if it were you in that situation? I think about that."

"No, why would I think that?" she recoiled.

It's really difficult to work in palliative care and not think about the end of your life. And caring for patients who are struggling makes me very grateful for what I have. Grateful for basic things that we often take for granted, like my ability to walk, to climb stairs, to make my bed, to wash my hair, and to cook something for myself.

THE FINANCIAL BURDEN OF FUNERALS

The financial burden of a funeral can sometimes shape a family's approach to end-of-life care for their loved one.

I've had relatives tell me they fear the judgment—by their community or religion or family—if they didn't have the money to give their family member a proper burial, and the situation was forcing them to keep someone on a ventilator instead of choosing palliative extubation.

"Right now, I don't have the money. So I'm not gonna make that decision right now. I have to wait until I get the money," they say.

LOIS

The drive through the winding streets of Floral Park is very enjoyable. I came upon the most beautiful street I had seen in a while. It was lined with sycamore trees, fully grown, with their branches intertwining in the sky across the two sides of the street like a natural wedding arch.

Lois lived in one of the unassuming houses on the street. She was a beautiful and smart lady who worked as a lobbyist. While she was working actively, she didn't pay much attention to her symptoms of bloating and constipation, figuring she was tired, overworked, and not eating right as a result. Then she went to her doctor and was diagnosed with advanced ovarian cancer, and it had spread throughout her entire abdomen. She was in shock at first, but being very practical and efficient, she quickly moved through the stages of grief.

When I visited her home as her hospice doctor, Lois cut to the chase. She said, "Just give me three good weeks. I need to tie up my work and get my affairs in order. That's all I need." We focused on fine tuning her medications and got her symptoms under control in two to three days. The hospice nurse reported back to our team that Lois was doing well, still working, and was meeting with her niece to arrange her affairs. We were all happy for her.

Exactly three weeks later, Lois died.

Even though I knew Lois was terminally ill, her death still came as a shock to me. She was so "stable" even though her disease was quite aggressive. I marveled at each person's knowledge of their body and the fact that Lois predicted her own destiny with such accuracy! I learned to really *listen* to patients' predictions of their life expectancy and not take these conversations for granted.

During those three weeks, Lois mapped out everything and didn't leave a single detail of her life to interpretation—including her funeral. It was her final assignment, and one she handled with the utmost professionalism and care.

MARIA

Maria was a social worker who worked in all settings of care, including hospital, home care, rehabilitation, school system, and others. She loved to read, write, and think. She also loved to entertain, play music, and talk to people.

She was diagnosed with end-stage pulmonary fibrosis, which is a progressive condition of the lungs in which they become scarred and unable to absorb oxygen. She knew eventually she would not be able to breathe, speak, or do much of anything else. Having counseled many clients and patients about funeral planning, Maria decided she would take things into her own hands. She wanted to plan a last party to host all her friends and say her goodbyes in lieu of her funeral. She believed that the eulogies should be presented to the person while she was alive rather than dead.

Maria got together with her close friends and family members and got to work, picking the music she wanted to play, the colors of the flowers she wanted to have, and the photos she wanted to show.

She lined up speakers who wanted to say something at her "funeral party" but told them she didn't want to know the content—she wanted to be surprised by what they had to say. At times, Maria felt unsure about this "live funeral" project, feeling vulnerable about what would happen and all that could go wrong.

But in the end, she decided, "What's the worst thing that could happen? I'm going to die?!"

This thought was so ridiculous that it made her laugh and stop worrying. Everything turned out beautifully, and her end-of-life party was one of her best memories.

HOMECOMING ("I WANT A LAVENDER COFFIN")

When I first introduced myself, Mrs. Johnson was very suspicious of my visit. She fired a series of questions at me:

- "Who are you?"
- "Are you going to stick me?"
- "Who told you to come?"
- "What'chu gonna do to me?"

Rose, her friend and caregiver, explained to Mrs. Johnson my role in overseeing her medical care as the hospice doctor, and that "Dr. Pan is on our side." Then Mrs. Johnson calmed down a bit.

Mrs. Johnson was a 95-year-old woman who, years earlier, had worked at a preeminent hospital in Manhattan and got to know all the doctors there. When she got sick, she always went to see the doctors "on the third floor" and never had to deal with any "clinic doctors." She was proud of her accomplishments and contributions.

We talked about Mrs. Johnson's husband—he had died decades earlier—and what she did after her retirement. Mrs. Johnson had been traveling around the world for many years, and her most memorable trip was "Christmas in Egypt" with Dr. Ben, a great African American philosopher. She reveled in her memories for a few moments with a faraway gaze. "I'll never forget that trip as long as I live!"

Rose smiled and explained, "Mrs. Johnson is the matriarch of the block! Everyone in the neighborhood loves her."

Mrs. Johnson eventually told me, "I know I will never be the same. But I will put one foot in front of the other and do the best I can."

When Rose stepped out, Mrs. Johnson told me that she asked Rose to find a local undertaker and instructed Rose to pick out a "lavender coffin" for her. She also told Rose that she wanted to be dressed up in a pink/lavender top and "look my best" for the homecoming.

MRS. KIM

Jane (my wonderful nursing colleague) and I visited Mrs. Kim in her hospital room. Mrs. Kim was always tranquil, quiet, and elegant, even as she lay in her hospital sick bed. Visiting her always reminded me of the busy fairy godmothers flitting around the princess. Her five daughters were always busying themselves about her, fixing her hair, straightening her blanket, adding a velvety robe from home, and moistening her lips.

The most impressive thing was that everything was pink. She loved pink, just like the actress Audrey Hepburn, who Mrs. Kim adored.

In addition to talking about medical treatment plans, we would discuss Mrs. Kim's experiences as a teacher, an advocate, and a guide to her daughters.

This family was not afraid to talk about Mrs. Kim's terminal illness, celebrate her last stage of life, and map out her funeral plans. When Mrs. Kim could not speak anymore due to her progressing illness, the planning came into focus.

They planned for a pink casket, pink flowers, a pink dress—pink everything.

I was amazed at the clarity they had and the dedication to Mrs. Kim's favorite color. It was a funeral fit for a movie star.

MY DAD

As I write this book, my own father faces multiple medical problems, and has become frailer, falls frequently, and is able to do less. Whereas in the past he avoided talking about end-of-life planning, now he is very open. He wrote out a simple will in Chinese and showed it to me and my brothers. He wrote that he did not want a funeral. He wished to be cremated and we could decide what to do about his ashes. Being his usual frugal self, he did not want to go to a lawyer and pay money to execute his will or to establish any kind of trust. Although it was sad for me to talk about his funeral, it was also a relief to know his thoughts, be able to listen to his wishes, and have a heart-to-heart conversation.

LESSONS

- Planning a funeral empowers you to face your own mortality, which can be scary. But it can also be calming and give someone a sense of purpose during a difficult time.
- Planning things out gives you control over what happens and helps relieve the burden on your family.
- Think about your preferences for your funeral if you wish to have one. Where would you hold it? Who would be involved? What music would play? Don't be afraid to actually plan your own funeral and hold it before you die. It might be fun!
- It can be so much easier to sort out your funeral details ahead of time instead of waiting for a time of crisis. Hospitals only keep bodies for two or three days after someone's death—but if you have even basic plans in place (such as the funeral home), it will make things so much easier for the deceased's relatives.

CHAPTER 16

Capacity

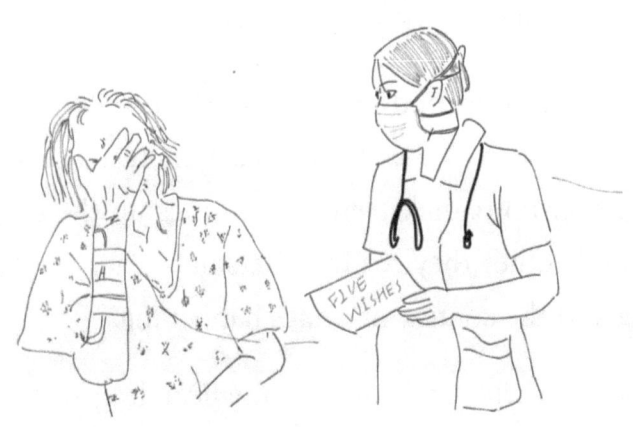

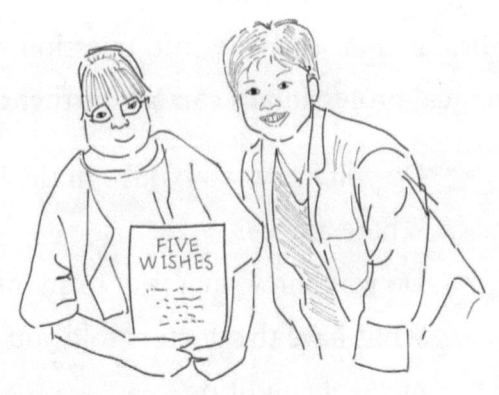

Exit Strategies

PALLIATIVE CARE PHYSICIANS ARE TASKED WITH assessing a patient's capacity for making decisions. Patients over the age of 18 are presumed to have mental capacity. When someone gets sick—or is diagnosed with dementia—and they're facing critical medical decisions, they are still assumed to have capacity until we start to question it.

Any time somebody has a change in their mental status—such as they begin to act confused or say things that don't make sense—it brings up the concern of whether they really understand what they're saying and the context of what's happening.

Can they truly make serious medical decisions?

If they're acting confused or delirious, saying things that don't necessarily make too much sense, it brings their capacity into question, st which point medical professionals can ask further questions:

- Do you know why you're in the hospital?
- Where are we?
- Do you know what year or month it is?
- What have the doctors told you about your medical condition?

Physicians can do an official assessment to test a patient's capacity. Two doctors have to concur that the patient has lost capacity to make certain decisions. If someone has lost capacity, major decisions instead will be discussed with the patient's healthcare proxy or surrogate decision-makers.

WHEN PATIENTS MASK THEIR DEMENTIA

Sometimes it's very difficult to tell if someone has lost capacity. This can be true with some dementia patients who are known to mask their problems well. People don't want others to know they have dementia and can't remember things. It's embarrassing and difficult.

I've had situations where a patient with dementia would answer questions in an abrasive or non-specific manner.

"Can you tell me where you are?" I'll ask.

"I'm here where everybody is. Where you are?" they say.

"Okay, can you tell me the name of this place?"

"It's the place. Don't you know the name?"

They're not answering the question, and that is usually a fair indication that they don't know. Sometimes people get offended by those questions, and I've had to tell them, "Listen, I don't mean to insult your intelligence or anything. We ask these questions routinely of all our patients, because there are decisions to be made, and we want to make sure that we are following your best interests."

TRYING TO UNDERSTAND A PATIENT'S CAPACITY

If we have patients who might have memory or capacity issues, one strategy we'll try is to have the patient sit in front and have their family sit behind them as we ask them a few questions.

"Do you take your own medications?" we ask.

The patient may say yes, and the family member behind them may shake their head no.

"Do you know what medications you're taking? Tell me the names of them."

"Well, there's the red one, the white one, and the blue one."

If a patient is in the hospital, or they're at a doctor's appointment, they should generally know their condition.

I'll say, "Tell me about your medical conditions," or "What's the reason you're in a hospital?" And sometimes, they don't know. That makes me worried.

CAPACITY VARIES BY THE DECISION

Decision-making capacity varies by the decision. Even if someone has moderate or severe dementia, they may still communicate effectively but lack good short-term memory. In this case, their proxy would make healthcare decisions instead. But the patient could still make lower-tier decisions for themselves, like the shirt they'd like to wear or what they'd like to eat for dinner. Meal choices are an easy decision, whereas the preference to use or not use a feeding tube, or whether someone wishes to be resuscitated, is much more complex. People need to be able to absorb complex information and understand the real risks versus the benefits in order to make such decisions.

RESEARCHING HEALTHCARE PROXY LAWS

We recommend that patients, while they have capacity, have a conversation about advanced directives and appoint a healthcare proxy to make medical decisions on their behalf, in case they lose the capacity to make their own decisions in the future..

We often ask why they chose one person over another to serve as their healthcare proxy—and their reasoning speaks to their capacity. If they want one person over another, that's a choice, and choices are good. Maybe one person has more medical experience. Or they live closer or is calmer than the other. It could be anything, and it shows their reasoning process. It is important to explain to your family that when you select one family member over another to serve as your "healthcare proxy," it doesn't mean you love them more. It just means that they may think more like you, know more about your medical condition, or are in a more suitable place to help you make medical decisions.

If they answer, "I don't know," that's an indication that they're not exhibiting reasoning and aren't able to explain their thought process. The more reasoning, the better. But sometimes we can't get that. Often, it's a process. It takes more than one conversation.

Some states have a healthcare proxy law. These states recognize the healthcare proxy as that extra-special person that was handpicked by the patient. Other states don't have that.

So if the patient now has no capacity to make complex medical decisions, and there is no healthcare proxy that was handpicked by the patient, then you go to next of kin. And every state has their rules about that as well.

You should research the laws around healthcare proxy in your state. You can use Google or ask your doctor or lawyer. Alternatively, you can use a document called Five Wishes (www.fivewishes.org/), which is an advance directive document that is accepted in the vast majority of U.S. states (except New Hampshire, Kansas, Ohio, or Texas) and is available in several languages.

In New York State, the Family Health Care Decisions Act (FHCDA)[10] outlines the correct course of action if there's no capacity and no proxy, and determines a hierarchy of decision-makers. Normally it begins with the legal guardian, followed by a spouse or domestic partner, and then by any adult children over the age of 18. After adult children comes parents, then brothers and sisters, and then other relatives and friends.

So you could have a situation where somebody has an intimate partner who isn't married and they don't necessarily live together, and on that hierarchy, that partner is last—even though they're probably the person who the patient would want to have making medical decisions for them.

Sometimes these situations can become very contentious.

---

10 Robert N. Swindler, "The Family Health Care Decisions Act: A Summary of Key Provisions," *NYSBA Health Law Journal* 15, no. 1 (2010), https://nysba.org/NYSBA/Public%20Resources/Family%20Healthcare%20Decisions%20Act%20Resource%20Center/FHDAC%20Files/SwidlerHealthJournSpr10.pdf.

CAPACITY FOR THOSE WITH INTELLECTUAL AND DEVELOPMENTAL DISABILITIES

I'm certified to assess capacity for patients who have intellectual and developmental disabilities, and I have special interest in that group because of my brother.

My brother, despite being 50 years old, has a mind that operates on a 10-year-old level because of his developmental disability. He's very smart in terms of knowing people and who he trusts and likes, and he has appointed me as his healthcare proxy. He makes a lot of decisions in his day-to-day life. But when the conversation turns to resuscitation and ventilation and feeding tubes and advance directives, it's too much for him to handle.

EXTRA LAYERS AND MEASURES

Patients with intellectual/developmental disabilities are a vulnerable population, and they endure additional measures when facing end-of-life care. In New York State, you cannot put in any orders to withdraw or withhold life-sustaining treatments (like cardiopulmonary resuscitation) for this population for at least 48 hours—you have to complete a checklist that specifies the end-of-life situation and terminal diagnosis, and a terminal diagnosis cannot be the developmental disorder.

Decisions can be put on hold for 48 hours, which can be a long time if the patient's medical situation is very unstable. Each step comes with extra layers of oversight. Every state may have different laws or regulations when it comes to this vulnerable patient population.[11]

WHAT YOU CAN DO

If you're worried because you or a loved one is struggling with any of these issues, it's important to raise that concern with your family or primary care doctor and get it investigated. In some cases, there could be other issues impacting a person's capacity, such as oxygen levels.

---

11 Caitlyn M. Moore et al., "Top Ten Tips Palliative Care Clinicians Should Know About Navigating the Needs of Adults with Intellectual Disabilities," *Journal of Palliative Medicine* 25, no. 12 (2022), 1857–1864. https://doi.org/10.1089/jpm.2022.0384.

Capacity

We always try to preserve the highest functioning the patient has—whatever they can do, we try to let them do that and not overly help them. The more you do for someone, the more they expect and the less they do on their own.

On top of that, you should find resources that can help the patient live the most independent life that they can.

> **LESSONS**
>
> - Patients over the age of 18 (in some states, over 19 years of age) are presumed to have mental capacity, including when facing serious illness.[12]
> - Patients with intellectual/developmental disabilities are a vulnerable population, and they endure additional measures when facing end-of-life care. They need their families and doctors to be their advocates!

---

12 "'Death with Dignity' Laws by State," FindLaw, last modified July 1, 2023, https://www.findlaw.com/healthcare/patient-rights/death-with-dignity-laws-by-state.html.

- Decision-making capacity varies by the decision. Even patients suffering from dementia can and should be able to make some decisions in their day-to-day lives.

CHAPTER 17

Sex in the City, at the End of Life

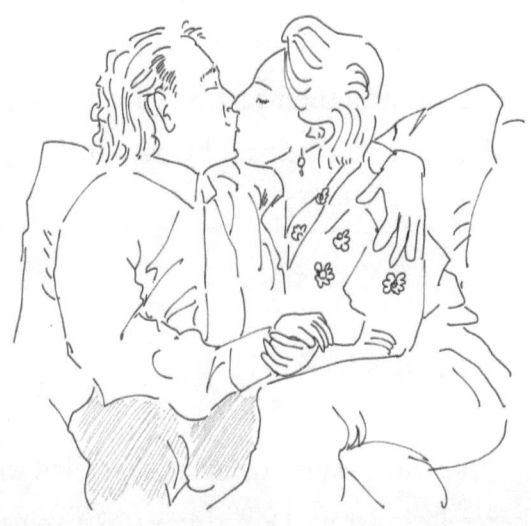

SEX IS ONE OF THE FEW TOPICS THAT'S AS uncomfortable for people to talk about as death.

When people are facing the end of their life, they tend to lose their filter and loosen up a bit. They feel a sense of freedom—the sense that they can say whatever they want. Perhaps they cannot control their feelings or are drudging up long-lost memories or flashbacks.

End-of-life care provides a window into people's lives.

As a result, there's a strange crossroads between these two topics—something I've discovered in caring for patients nearing the end of their life. To me, these sexual comments and situations reflect the essence of who the patients and their relatives are and what lives they've led, and it can help to bring a little lightness of being.

DOROTHY AND RON

Dorothy and Ron were what they called a May-December relationship. Dorothy was 20 years older than Ron. They met at a local bar in Jackson Heights, New York. From what I understood, they used to be bar buddies together and were quite a jovial couple.

By the time I met her, Dorothy was in her late 70s and suffering from late-stage emphysema from her years of puffing smoke. She was able to sit in a chair but needed help getting there. She also needed help with urination and bathing.

I remember vividly the first time I saw her during a hospice home visit. She required Ron's help to clean her, and how clumsy he was at taking care of her. I remember my thought bubble, "Uh-oh, he's in trouble. I don't know how long she'll last at home. He'll probably be looking for a nursing home real soon."

The next time I visited Dorothy at home, she had declined significantly and was mainly in bed. She was becoming confused, and Ron was worried. I examined Dorothy, answered Ron's questions, and allayed his fears. When I introduced myself, her expression told me that she did not remember me.

Being a geriatrician, I asked her questions to test her memory and determine how oriented she was to her surroundings. When I asked her what year it was, she gave me a blank look. I then pointed to Ron who was standing at the foot of the hospital bed, and asked Dorothy, "Do you know who that gentleman is?"

She glanced at him and beamed, "That's my luvah!"

At first, I was shocked. I didn't know how to respond. At the same time, I felt like giving her a high five!

Could practicing medicine be any more fun than this?

I looked at Ron, who was also beaming from ear to ear. I told Ron, "She remembers the important things!"

This sweet moment lasted a couple of minutes, then Dorothy needed to be changed. Ron stepped right up. With skill, precision, and efficiency, he turned Dorothy part way, cleaned her with a wipe, massaged some A&D ointment on her buttocks, then returned her to a comfortable position.

My thought bubble this time was, "My goodness, he has grown so much as a caregiver. She is going to be all right after all."

FIJI AND FRANK

Fiji Majevski was a 90-year-old woman with end-stage ovarian cancer. She was quickly declining, becoming weaker, staying in bed more, and was not able to do things around the house. She lived with her husband, 92-year-old Frank. They had been married for 60 years and depended on each other for their daily activities.

But now that Fiji was bedbound, Frank was not able to give her physical care, such as bathing, changing, and cleaning after her bowel movements and urine. Every week when the nurse visited, Frank would ask her about "alternative treatments" and searched for another experimental treatment.

We all understood that Frank must be grief stricken. After all, his wife of 60-plus years was dying of cancer. Alternatively, perhaps at the advanced age of 92, Frank might not really remember that he was asking the same questions week after week.

The team asked me to visit them at home and answer some of the questions.

When I entered Fiji's room, Frank followed me in, appearing somewhat disheveled in a rumpled suit. I sat down at a chair next to Fiji's bedside to talk to her. She appeared pale and fatigued. She turned in toward the wall, and though she was not very interactive, she did allow me to examine her. I found a large mass and fluid in her abdomen. These were ominous findings.

After my examination, I asked Fiji if she had any questions for me, and she shook her head. I covered her back up and stood.

Frank followed me out to the living room.

"Doctor," he said, "is she getting better?"

"What do you think is going on with your wife, Mr. Majevski?" I reflected.

"Doctor, I really need my wife to get better. I just cannot lose her," Frank said in a shaky voice. "We are very close."

He moved closer to me, pointed downward with his arthritis-crippled index finger, and whispered, "Doctor, *my thing* won't go down. What am I to do?"

I looked at him in silence to buy time for my response. At the same time, I also edged my way toward the door, just in case I needed a swift getaway.

After I explored with Frank what medicines he was taking, I decided none of his meds were the culprit.

"Do you want my advice, Frank?" I asked.

"Yes, Doctor, please tell me what I can do," Frank urged.

"I'm afraid you will have to use your hands, sir."

"Oh, okay."

I said goodbye and made my swift getaway. As I stepped into my car, I gave myself a high five. "That was not a bad answer, Cynthia!"

STANLEY AND ROSE

Stanley and Rose lived in an enormous house in a beautiful section of Forest Hills Gardens, New York. They had no children but enjoyed their lives with each other, traveling frequently. Stanley had end-stage heart disease and peripheral vascular disease, and his toes were rotting away. I came to visit him at home along with his hospice nurse Jane so that we could make a wound care plan for his necrotic toes.

As we pulled up, Rose greeted us at the door. She led us through the serpentine halls into his bedroom.

Stanley was in bed, motionless. His longtime male aide, Carl, was sitting at his bedside. Jane and I put down our medical bags. I approached the bed and introduced myself.

"Mr. Stanley, my name is Dr. Pan. How are you doing today?"

No answer. Not even a blink.

After another attempt, Jane and I decided to move on and examine his feet and toes. Rose pulled out a rolling cart filled with wound care supplies. Carl helped Jane undress the dressing around Stanley's toes. I admired the rows of photos lining the walls, telling stories of the couple's years of traveling.

After looking at his toes and examining his circulation, Jane and I made a plan for Stanley's wound care. I returned to the head of the bed and made another attempt at engaging Stanley. I gently shook his shoulder and called out to him.

"Mr. Stanley, how are you feeling right now?"

Stanley opened his eyes a slit, and mouthed the words, *"When was the last time you were spanked."*

I nearly fell off my feet! "Did he just say what I thought he said?"

Maybe I wasn't so good at reading lips. I looked at Jane and Rose for help. Jane shrugged her shoulders and tried not to laugh. Carl chimed in. "Yup, that's what he said."

I didn't know what to say, so I replied, "Stanley, that's a *very* personal question."

Rose apologized. "I'm sorry. Stan always says that to the nurses!"

JOE

Joe was dying at home. His advanced cancer robbed him of all his energy. This was a devastating thing for a lively Italian guy who was usually the life of the party.

When I went to visit him at home, he was lying quietly across the sofa in the center of the living room. On another sofa sat his three brothers who stared forward with intense expressions.

His wife was cooking in the kitchen. I waved hello and introduced myself. The brothers nodded and pointed me to the kitchen. I went into the kitchen to speak with Joe's wife, who told me that Joe has been sleeping deeply since yesterday and not responding to her call. She then called his brothers, who came to see him.

After getting more history, I went to the sofa to talk to Joe. He was in a quiet, delirious state—not awake or alert, and not responding to my attempts to wake him. I touched Joe on the shoulder and gently shook him as I called his name. Still no response.

I shook him some more and said, "Joe, how are you? My name is Dr. Pan. I'm visiting you at home. Wake up, please." No response.

After another attempt, Joe opened his eyes and moaned in delirium. "Cheat on me, don't leave me."

Not expecting this response, I looked around. The three brothers sat still as his wife continued cooking in the kitchen.

LESSONS

- When people are facing the end of their life, they tend to lose their filter and feel a sense of freedom. Sexual innuendos and thoughts can be prominent.
- End-of-life care offers a window into people's lives, including their sexuality.
- Sexual comments bring a little surprise and twist and lighten up end-of-life conversations! It's okay to have these conversations!

CHAPTER 18

You Are My Final Doctor

IT WAS A CHILLY BUT SUNNY DAY IN MARCH. THE earth was awakening and spring was just around the corner, waiting to jumpstart life again. With my papers in hand, I went to visit a hospice patient.

Samuel Bradley was 94 years old and receiving hospice care for end-stage heart failure. He had two sons who lived out of state. Since he was now frail and homebound, he elected to have me (the hospice medical director) take over his medical care.

According to the hospice social worker, Samuel had been very vocal about his illness, speaking often about his life achievements and regrets, and expressing how at peace he was with dying. This behavior, in hospice language, is called "life review."

As I drove up to their house, a man in his 60s opened the door. I parked my car, took out my doctor's bag, and went to meet him. He had grayed hair, a gentle smile, and a meek manner.

"My name is Dr. Pan, and you are?" I asked.

"I'm Bob, Sam's son. I don't live here. I'm here from Montana, but I'm staying for a while until things get more settled with my dad."

"Why don't we talk a little bit in the living room before we see your dad?"

"Okay," replied Bob.

I took out my chart and began asking him about Sam's past medical history, the events that led up to his recent hospitalization, test results, and conversations that took place in the hospital. Pretty soon it became apparent that Bob had minimal information.

"My brother and I are trying to take turns being here. It's not very easy since we live so far away and have to juggle our own schedules. We tried to persuade him to move in with one of us, but he doesn't want to," he said.

"I hear you. It's very common for older people to not want to move from their homes," I said. "Why don't we go see your dad?"

Bob stood up and led me down the hallway, past the bathroom, and then to the bedroom. We walked into Samuel's room, which was bright and airy. He was finishing up breakfast from a bedside tray. He looked visibly emaciated and was receiving oxygen through his nose.

"Good morning, Mr. Bradley," I said. "My name is Dr. Pan."

"What?!" he said loudly.

"Good morning, Mr. Bradley. My name is Dr. Pan," I repeated, louder this time. "I'm from hospice care."

"Oh, Dr. Pan," he paused, then signaled for me to sit down in a chair next to him. He looked at me intently, then said, "That means you're my FINAL doctor."

Whooommmph! I felt like I was in a *Matrix* movie. Mr. Smith had just punched me in the chest and the force thrusted me a hundred feet away! In *slooooooooooooooow motion.*

I tried to compose myself, as no one had ever said that to me before even though I had visited hundreds of terminally ill patients. Bob looked visibly tense as he sat on the edge of the bed. Mr. Bradley, on the other hand, calmly took a sip of his morning tea.

"I guess so," I replied weakly.

"Well, give it to me straight. How long have I got?" demanded Mr. Bradley.

"Mr. Bradley, you don't mince words, do you?" I said in amazement. Bob was appearing more nervous. A brief silence took place. I said, "Well, I need some more information from the hospital. Like the echo-cardiogram result."

"Yes," confirmed Mr. Bradley. "They did do an echo."

"Yes, the echo. It's called the ejection fraction. It's usually a number—a percent."

"Ah," he declared. "The ejector fraction." I smiled. After a brief pause, he continued. "It's very bad. It's fifteen percent."

"That is pretty low," I confirmed.

"Well?" said Mr. Bradley, staring at me intensely.

"Well, given that ejection fraction and what's been happening with you, I would say a few months. Also, the fact that they recommended hospice for you means that the doctors at the hospital thought you probably had less than six months."

"All right. I won't put you on the hook." Mr. Bradley sat back understandingly. He then changed the topic.

"Where are you from? What country?"

"I'm Chinese American," I replied. We proceeded to talk about China—he had been there to visit and enjoyed Beijing and Shanghai. He talked about other travels with his wife and how he served as a Navy pilot in the war. He volunteered how grateful he felt for having the means to hire a private caregiver without having to overburden his family.

"What concerns or worries are on your mind?" I asked.

"I'm not afraid of dying. I've lived a very full life. I just don't want to go to the hospital again. I want to stay here until I die." Mr. Bradley outlined simply but elegantly his goals of care.

"I think that we can help you achieve that goal. We will do our best to treat you at home so that you are comfortable," I said earnestly.

"When are you coming again?" he asked, visibly fatigued.

"Whenever you want me to. Just tell your nurse, and she will let me know. It will be my pleasure." I said goodbye to Mr. Bradley and Bob led me back out into the hallway.

"I can't believe he said all those things!" Bob said.

"I know. I think your father is an amazing human being. It's really my honor to know him," I replied.

A GOOD THING OR A BAD THING?

After leaving Mr. Bradley's house, I sat in my car for quite a while, immobilized by his words. "You are my *final* doctor."

It was a big comment. I never thought of myself as "The Final Doctor." And I didn't know what to think about his comment. Was it a good thing? A bad thing? Was this what I signed up to do? Was this what I was meant to do?

Perhaps I should become a hospitalist instead.

It took me several days to process and reflect upon my practice. I realized that I loved what I did. Practicing hospice and palliative care is not for sissies. It takes courage, attention to detail, seeing the big picture, the ability to navigate conflicts and mediate difficult conversations, bear witness, and to acknowledge and reduce suffering. It's not something that every doctor can do. I happen to love it and be good at it. So why not me?

REVISITING WITH MR. BRADLEY

A few weeks after my visit with Mr. Bradley, I received an update about this care. He was becoming more short of breath, having pain, and staying in bed most of the time. We increased the amount of oxygen, made medication changes, and updated his sons about his decline.

I went back to visit Mr. Bradley upon his request. I drove up to the familiar street and house, parked my car, and rang the doorbell. A middle-aged woman—Mr. Bradley's privately hired caregiver, Marla—answered the door.

"I'm so glad you're here, doctor," Marla said. "Mr. Bradley is having a rough day."

We walked into the house and headed for Mr. Bradley's room. The room was dark, and I could hear the humming of the oxygen concentrator. Mr. Bradley was in the hospital bed. He was visibly thinner than the last time I saw him, which I did not think was possible. He grimaced and I noticed that it seemed difficult for him to breathe.

I greeted him. "Mr. Bradley. It's me—Dr. Pan. Do you remember me?"

He looked at me and smiled weakly. "Of course I do."

"Are you having pain?" I inquired.

"Yes. All over."

"Is it mild pain or pretty bad?"

"Bad," Mr. Bradley whispered.

"Do you want to take some pain medication?" I asked.

"Yes," he replied.

I turned to Marla and asked for Roxanol, the liquid morphine intensol that is very effective for the relief of pain and air hunger. Marla moved to the other side of the room to get the bottle. I asked Marla how much morphine Mr. Bradley had been using in the past two days. Marla brought over a notebook. Its pages were neatly lined with columns and had written notations of dates, times, and amount of medication taken. I scanned the log quickly and learned that each day he had been using the Roxanol at least seven times—either for pain or air hunger. He had received a dose about two hours prior to my arrival but was obviously still in pain and struggling to breathe. I instructed Marla to draw up an amount that was double the dose that Mr. Bradley had been receiving, and she gave it to him under the tongue.

Exit Strategies

As we waited for the medication to take effect, I examined Mr. Bradley. His blood pressure was borderline low, his lungs were congested, and his breathing was noisy. His abdomen felt somewhat distended, and he reported constipation. Thanks to Marla's meticulous care, Mr. Bradley did not have any pressure ulcers or bed sores.

I reviewed Mr. Bradley's medication list and found he was still taking his usual three cardiac medications, which could be lowering his blood pressure excessively. He was also taking his cholesterol pill even though he'd lost 30 pounds and was not eating very much each day. As a result, his cholesterol level was now normal.

"I will be changing your medications today," I told Mr. Bradley. "You do not need all these medications. Do you want me to call your son?"

"Yes, and please tell Marla. Marla is my lifesaver," Mr. Bradley nodded.

"How is your pain now?" I followed up.

"Much better. My breathing too." Mr. Bradley was able now to speak in longer phrases since his symptoms were better controlled.

I sat down in the chair next to Mr. Bradley's bed and started writing down the medication changes in the logbook. When visiting patients who are elderly and very sick, it's crucial to review their medications carefully during each visit. As patients' medical conditions change, their medications need to be adjusted to account for their functional status, nutritional status, kidney function, and goals of care.

I've learned that with medications, "Less is more." Does it make any sense to continue giving a patient like Mr. Bradley cholesterol medication when he's a skeleton and hardly eating? Many cholesterol medications can also cause musculoskeletal pain, and it was my determination that this could be contributing to his increase in pain. Similarly, he'd been on three cardiac medications. But now his heart disease was at the end stage and his blood pressure was running low. We needed to re-evaluate his heart medications to balance their risks and benefits.

Because Mr. Bradley has been bedbound, eating and drinking little, and taking morphine for pain, he was constipated and at risk for fecal impaction.

He needed to have a good bowel regimen to keep his bowel movements going.

I finished writing the changes to his medications and decided to stop one cardiac medication and decrease the dose of the other. I increased the dosage of Mr. Bradley's morphine based on how much he needed. I also increased his laxatives to give him more effective bowel movements.

I left the room to call Bob to review the med changes and the reasons for doing so. Bob was very grateful for my visit and the information and said his brother Bill was coming next week. When I was about to hang up, Bob asked nervously, "How long do you think he has?" It turns out Bob had been trying to rearrange his schedule to visit Mr. Bradley and wanted to know when he should come.

"I'm seeing that he's declining steadily," I told Bob. "It may only be on the order of weeks. You should come sooner rather than later."

"What is the end like? Will he have a lot of pain?"

"He is already having increasing pain and shortness of breath. These are very common symptoms in end-stage heart failure. I've made adjustments to his meds, and we will keep assessing him and make changes as needed to ensure he's comfortable at home. As we know, his goal is to stay at home and not return to the hospital. We can help him achieve that goal," I reassured Bob. "Also, you should feel free to call us any time, 24/7. If you have any questions or concerns or want to talk face to face when you are here, let me know and I will make a visit."

"Okay, thank you so much!"

A REWARDING ROLE

After leaving Mr. Bradley's house, I sat in my car for quite a while. I reflected on the words he'd spoken earlier, and what they meant to me: "You are my *final* doctor."

For many in my profession, being someone's *final doctor* is not why we chose this career path. Seeing patients die is not easy, and dealing with the emotions and family dynamics can be draining. Yet, we are here to help our patients and families navigate through some of the toughest times in their lives. We are present with them through this end-of-life journey and help them grow and push beyond their comfort zones.

How meaningful and rewarding it was to be his final doctor.

LESSONS

- Be nice to your final doctor!
- Be open to conducting your own "Life Review"—talk about your achievements, regrets, memorable moments! Sharing is caring.
- Be open and upfront with your palliative care team about your goals, needs, and wishes.
- Being someone's final doctor is probably not the reason why your doctor pursued a career in medicine—but they are in that role because they want to help people like you at your time of need.

CHAPTER 19

Discussing Advance Directives with My Parents and Brother

TALKING ABOUT ADVANCE DIRECTIVES ISN'T easy for any family—even mine.

After decades of discussing advance directives with my patients, I realized that I never had these important conversations with my parents or brother, the latter of which has intellectual/developmental disabilities (I/DD). Armed with all my experiences, I thought this would be easy-peasy. Right?

DAD

I decided to broach the topic during a visit to my parents' house in Flushing, Queens.

Exit Strategies

My dad was sitting in the living room watching Chinese CCTV while my mom was in the kitchen making a nice cup of green tea and bringing out snacks. I sat down in the living room and had a casual conversation with my dad—we talked about the weather and what was happening in China, Taiwan, and Hong Kong.

During a break from the chitchat, I steered the conversation toward advance directives.

"Have you ever heard of advance directives?" I asked. Silence. The TV was loud.

I continued, "You know, to talk about your wishes in advance, in case you get so sick later and cannot tell us your wishes."

I could feel the room tense up. It felt like the temperature might have dropped a few degrees. As the TV announcer talked about controversies between Taiwan and China, I could sense friction brewing in the room. My dad looked away from the TV, his brow furrowed, and responded. "You know, after I die, one-third of everything will go to you. So you don't have to rush it."

Dad got up and went upstairs. The hairs on my neck bristled, and I thought, "Oh man, that did *not* go well."

MOM

A few minutes later, my mom came in from the kitchen to check on us.

"Where's dad?" she asked.

"He went upstairs," I said. "Have a seat, mom. Get some rest."

Mom sat down next to me on the sofa with her tea.

"What's going on? How is your work?" she asked.

"Tough. Lots of patients without advance directives. When they get sick, their families don't know what they want or what to do." I asked my mom, "Have you ever heard of advance directives?"

"I'm not sure," Mom replied.

"Well, it's basically talking about your wishes in advance, what's important to you, before you get very sick—sometimes so sick that you cannot express yourself or tell us your wishes. It's a good idea, even though it's hard to talk about."

"Oh, that sounds very scary," Mom commented.

Fortunately, Mom cooperated with me. She stayed in the room, listened to my questions, and told me about her preferences for when "the time comes," if she were at the end of life and could not speak for herself. She expressed how much she valued things like being independent, cooking, playing sudoku, going out to lunch with her friends, visiting the senior center to learn new activities (such as drawing, painting, singing, and calligraphy), and spending time with her family. She would not want to be in a vegetative state and linger on machines. She would want to have a trial of critical care if this could make her recover and bring her back to living at home independently.

PETER

As I spoke to my mother, my brother Peter was present.

Discussing Advance Directives with My Parents and Brother

The topic of conversation made me think back to when we were growing up and our dad would jokingly ask Peter, "Who would you want to go live with after we (mom and dad) die?"

Peter's answer was always, "Number One." He wouldn't call me by my name but rather "Number One" because I am the oldest born and he is the youngest (Number Three). Peter did not always get along with our middle brother, Number Two. When my dad asked Peter about living with our middle brother, or being cared for by him, Peter would adamantly decline.

After Mom told us what was important to her, I asked Peter if all this made sense to him. It astonished me when Peter held his head with both hands and screamed, "Can you stop talking about this? It's making my head hurt!"

It was a reminder of the nuances involved with capacity—Peter is capable of appointing a healthcare proxy but lacks the capacity to make complex medical decisions. Even talking about those what-if situations made his head hurt.

IMPORTANT LESSONS

I reflected on the conversation with my dad and what went wrong in the days that followed. I realized that my approach might have been too direct—which, as I learned from reviewing medical literature, isn't advisable with Chinese persons. Being too direct can be perceived as bringing on a bad omen and being disrespectful. I also did not introduce the topic well or give him a context of why this conversation was important.

I could see how he might have been confused about my intent—his mind immediately went to money, thinking that was my reason for asking.

The awkwardness and difficulty in having that conversation with my father hammered home the reality that people often aren't comfortable talking about advance directives and put off the conversation for as long as they can. But as I knew far too well, putting off that conversation too long could lead to suffering and confusion.

It gave me appreciation for my patients and their families who, at my urging, found a way to talk about advance directives. Being on the other side of the equation wasn't easy, even with all of my palliative care experience.

TAKING A DIFFERENT APPROACH

I tried a different tack the next time I visited my parents. As I walked to the grocery store with my dad, he asked me about my work. I vented about how hard my work was, talking about the very sick ICU patient that I was seeing that week.

His immediate question was "How old is he?" I responded that the patient was about his age, which piqued his interest.

"What happened to him?" Dad pressed on. I described that the patient was elderly, came from home, had high blood pressure, heart disease, and pulmonary COPD, and came to the hospital for bad pneumonia.

"How bad was the pneumonia? Was it as bad as the one I had a couple of years ago?"

"Yes, much worse. Because of this acute illness, he went into respiratory failure and needed to be intubated. He went to the ICU and became confused and agitated. He tried to pull out the tube going from his throat/airway to the machine, but the nurses put mittens on his hands so he couldn't grab anything. Then his kidneys failed and the ICU doctors put another catheter to dialyze him. Then he got more confused." I could see my dad was aghast.

"If that happened to me, I would just shoot myself," he said.

"You don't have a gun, do you?"

"No, but I wouldn't like that. If I can't walk around, plant winter melons in my garden, travel back and forth to China, or speak for myself, then that's it."

"What do you mean 'that's it'?"

"That would not be a good way to live anymore. Who wants to live like that?!"

Discussing Advance Directives with My Parents and Brother

I was grateful for this conversation. At least now I felt like I have a more solid idea of what mattered to my dad—a proud, strong, dignified man who used to be a diplomat. Sometimes—whether because of a person's age, customs, or cultural norms—they might not be comfortable discussing advance directives head-on, but you can gather insights about their thinking by asking them hypotheticals and seeing how they respond. One example could be the case of Terri Schiavo, or one of the many of the other examples in this book that could be used an icebreaker to start this important conversation. Remember, these conversations evolve over time. Do not expect it to be completed in one sitting.

HELPFUL TIPS ON STARTING THE CONVERSATION

Use any excuse you can to start this meaningful conversation with yourself and your loved ones. You can preface the discussion by saying, "This is not a comfortable conversation, yet it's very important." Ease into the conversation by mentioning how you heard something on the news. Or happened to read a book—like this one. Maybe you could mention how you listened to a podcast on the topic, or how somebody was talking to you about it. Use an example from the COVID-19 pandemic, or if you're a *Seinfeld* fan, you could've watched the episode where Kramer (played by Michael Richards) decides to draw up a living will after watching a movie about a woman in a coma, and chooses Elaine (Julia Louis Dreyfus) as his executor. At first, he wants to forgo life support—but later changes his mind after watching the rest of the movie.

Find a way into the conversation that feels natural and logical, and start the conversation slowly. Plant the seeds, then water and fertilize them by following up on the conversation later. Remember, the person you're speaking with is probably not going to be ready and may feel unsettled or uncomfortable about the topic. Your goal is to make them feel more comfortable about it.

If somebody reacts the wrong way, don't take it personally—it's their fear response. They'd rather not think about the end of their life, and who can blame them? It's like the *New York Times* cartoonist, Roz

Chast, who wrote her graphic memoir, *Can't We Talk About Something More Pleasant?*, depicting her experiences caregiving for her elderly parents.[13]

Don't be discouraged, and don't give up! The conversation gets easier. Trust me! But somebody has to start the conversation.

Why not you?

TALKING WITH MEDICAL PROFESSIONALS

Once you start the conversation with your loved ones, it's important to continue that conversation with medical professionals.

Surveys[14] show that medical professionals think advance directives are important, but they often wait for patients to start the conversation, as they worry about making patients nervous or unsettled. Patients, meanwhile, find advance directives important as well,

---

13   Roz Chast, *Can't We Talk About Something More Pleasant?* (New York: Bloomsbury Publishing, 2014).
14   Terry Fulmer et al., "Physicians' Views on Advance Care Planning and End-of-Life Care Conversations," *Journal of the American Geriatrics Society* 66, no. 6 (2018): 1201–1205, https://doi.org/10.1111/jgs.15374.

but aren't likely to discuss them with their physicians.[15] Unless the doctors ask.

Everybody, it seems, wants somebody else to start the conversation. In my family's case, I visited my father's primary care physician and reminded the doctor to bring up the topic.

DOCUMENTATION

The doctor, thankfully, did follow up—and gave my parents and brother healthcare proxy forms to complete.

A couple of weeks later, Peter and my parents came over to my house for a family get-together. My mom pulled a bunch of documents out of her tote, saying, "Our doctor wants us to fill out these proxies. We don't know how to do it, but we know you do!"

Wow! Even if things were tense at the onset, my family had come so far in being able to discuss their

---

[15] Rory O'Sullivan et al., "Advance Directives: Survey of Primary Care Patients," *Canadian Family Physician (Medecin De Famille Canadien)* 61, no. 4 (2015), 353–356.

advance directives. It was a reminder of how important it is for everyone to row the boat in the same direction. In this situation, it was important for my family to trust me and continue this conversation, for their primary care doctor to support this advance directives conversation, and for me to not give up and continue to find out what matters most to my family.

PEACE OF MIND

AFTER FACING MY FATHER'S RESISTANCE WHEN I first brought up advance directives, the conversation has gotten easier and easier since then. I came across a Chinese book about a famous Chinese writer who had to advocate for her husband's wishes not to receive an artificial feeding tube at the end of life. I brought it to my parents' house and raved about it. A few weeks later, my dad commented to me about how he read the book and completely agreed with the writer. Dad said, "Make sure you don't put a feeding tube in me if I ever get so sick and cannot recover."

I was shocked about how openly Dad was talking about his wishes and preferences, especially after the initial resistance.

Following a recent surgery, Dad told me, "You know, I've had a great life with wonderful children. I have no regrets. And when I die, I want you to cremate me, and then I want you to take your boat out and spread my ashes all over the water."

It's been so powerful for me to be able to talk to my relatives and find out their wishes—it's given all of us so much peace of mind.

Believe me—by starting the conversation, you can help to diminish the stigmas around advance directives and give permission to have these important conversations!

LESSONS

- If you start a conversation about advance directives with your family, ease into it by using any excuse you can to begin the conversation—whether it's a news story, a TV show, or even this book! If they are ready to talk about this

topic, great. If they're not comfortable, don't push them—you can bring it up another time.
- Don't be afraid to start the conversation with your doctor, too, and fill out the necessary forms. Talk to them about what brings you meaning and joy, what makes your life worth living, and what makes your life not worth living.
- Discuss advance directives *in advance*, and don't wait until the last minute or for a crisis to happen. Many people who do not start these conversations regret it later.
- Keep in mind that as we grow and age, our opinions and goals may change. That's okay too.

CHAPTER 20

The EOL Passport for Our Last Journey

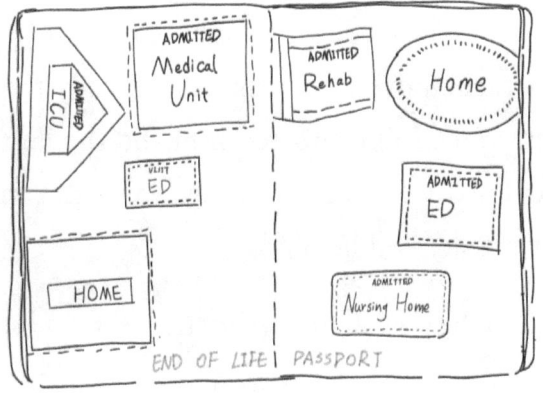

DOCTORS TYPICALLY GO INTO MEDICINE TO HELP people—to *save* and *cure* everybody.

Oh, how noble, and how naive. The minute you go into medicine, you have to face the reality: some patients are inevitably going to die. And maybe it will be up to you to tell their families the bad news.

Exit Strategies

I didn't sign up for that, you might think.

I was a medical student when my first patient died. He was a sweet, elderly man admitted for heart failure. I formed a good rapport with him and had great conversations with him when the residents and attending doctors were too busy to speak at length.

On that fateful day, I heard the overhead pager call, "Code Blue, Code Blue," and it was my patient's room! I rushed over; my team was already there. We administered CPR, intubated him, did the best chest compressions we could, and gave him the medications available. And he died.

I fled to the on-call room, shut the door, and sobbed.

My resident doctor knocked on the door and said, "Cynthia, his family is here. Do you want to tell them what happened?" I curled up in the room.

"No, no—you tell them," I said through tears.

Those conversations are never easy—and I think I chose palliative care as a career, in part, so I could develop the courage to walk up to a patient's family, tell them how much I appreciated knowing their family member, and how bad I feel for their loss.

Through these tough conversations, I've learned how to talk to people and provide some form of comfort in the most difficult situations. Sometimes it is best to not say anything at all. Just sit, allow the silence to take over, and be present.

It's why I teach courses for other medical professionals about end-of-life conversations and the motivation behind writing this book. I want all of us to be better prepared to have these difficult conversations, and I want patients and their family members to feel better prepared for their medical journey.

DR. PELLEGRINO'S EXAMPLE

People react differently as the end of their life approaches. Some people expand out and connect with everybody—they want to touch the whole world. Others shrink away and hide.

Exit Strategies

Some are open about their prognosis, like former president Jimmy Carter, who announced to the country that he chose to enroll in hospice care at home! Others face their health challenges silently, privately.

Some want to know every detail about what's to come. Some want to hear only general information. Others don't want to know anything.

How you approach EOL care is a personal choice! I draw so much inspiration from those who are open about their circumstances. One of those people is Dr. Thomas Pellegrino, a leader in neurology and medical ethics, who served as an associate dean for education at Eastern Virginia Medical School.[16]

In 2011, Dr. Pellegrino was diagnosed with a terminal illness. Instead of retreating into his own world, he decided to make his diagnosis widely known and use his situation as a teaching case. He welcomed students and other people to speak to him and was open about his experiences as a patient. He also wrote a series of four letters that served as the basis of a learning series.

---

16   "Dr. Thomas R. Pellegrino," *Virginian Pilot*, Legacy.com, accessed January 23, 2024, https://www.legacy.com/us/obituaries/pilotonline/name/thomas-pellegrino-obituary?id=26116244.

I was honored to participate in a presentation about therapeutic listening centered around distilling what matters most to our patients who went through experiences similar to Dr. Pellegrino's. My session was a fireside chat about his second letter that discussed the topic "what matters most." I love that topic.

Far too often, patients, their family members, and their doctors have very different goals. What's important for a patient is not always important for their doctor. The letters reinforced the need for patients to be clear about their wishes—and for medical workers to ask the right questions.

More than a decade after Dr. Pellegrino's death, his impact and legacy live on.

A STRANGE TRIP TO A STRANGE PLACE

I love traveling! And in a lot of ways, end-of-life care resembles a trip—I liken healthcare transfers as trips to exotic places where you may not know the people, the language, or the culture.

Exit Strategies

When a patient arrives at the hospital, they get processed in the system and get a wristband, and that's like stamping your passport. Now you get moved up to the medical surgical unit. Now it's a different team. It's like you're going into a different country—you get another stamp.

Something happens and your condition worsens, and you go to the ICU (intensive care unit). Another stamp and another country.

The culture and languages in each of these places differ. Cardiologists speak one language, while the nurses and palliative care doctors speak another. Sometimes you can pick up pieces of the conversation, and other times it's completely foreign—which can be so confusing.

Patients and family members often want to ask for instructions, but they don't want to appear like they don't belong, so they stay quiet.

My mother sent me a saying that really encapsulates the feelings around end-of-life care and our personal journeys: "We are all tourists and God is our travel agent who already fixed all our routes, reservations, and destinations. So, trust Him and *enjoy the trip called life."*

PREPARING FOR A TRIP

How do you go about preparing for a trip? Maybe you read about the place and check reviews from previous visitors. You plan an itinerary and figure out what to pack. You decide who you want to take the trip, the ways to stay in touch with your loved ones, and prepare emergency contact information if something goes wrong. And while on your trip, you should know at least a little bit of the local language.

In my opinion, our preparations for end-of-life care should follow a similar path. It helps to have your plans sorted out and a healthcare proxy appointed just in case.

SPEAKING THE RIGHT LANGUAGE

Doctors, nurses, and medical institutions can also do a better job of communicating with patients and their families in ways that can be more easily understood.

I realized early on that when I speak medical language with my patients, their eyes glaze over.

For example, doctors have to write a "chief complaint" in the chart to describe the main reason why patients came to the hospital or the clinic. Well, I was rounding in the ICU as a resident and a whole group of us went to see a patient. I asked, "Mr. Smith, what complaints do you have today?"

Mr. Smith rushed to explain. "Oh no, I don't complain, doctor. I'm a very good patient."

Another example is in medical school while I was caring for surgery patients. We all had to write admitting orders that included Is and Os—which stand for Inputs and Outputs. Input equals what patients take in orally or via intravenous fluids, and Output equals what patients excrete or otherwise put out. As a new student, my resident directed me to write orders for Is and Os. What I ended up writing was "eyes and nose."

If a medical student could make these mistakes, what are patients to do?

TRAINS, BOATS, AND AUTOMOBILES

Since we're talking end of life as a journey, we need to discuss modes of transportation.

Our bodies are fantastic, amazing, intricately made modes of transportation. Our bodies are made to move and take us on journeys and voyages. Even when people are born with disabilities or become injured, they still find ways to move. Think of the Paralympic athletes!

When people stop moving, they are in trouble! The old adage of "use it or lose it" is true. We cannot and should not take our bodies and mobility for granted. This is a call for everyone out there to go out and move it! Use whatever type of movement or exercise you like. It could be walking, strolling, running, Zumba, aerobics, swimming, treadmill, biking, dancing, housework, push-ups, sit-ups—whatever you like. But you must do it and do it consistently. There's great research that shows that consistent exercise and movements lead to better health, less chronic illnesses, and more longevity!

With aging and wear and tear, our bodies begin to break down. Yet we adjust, slow down, expect less, and learn to use adaptive equipment like canes, crutches, walkers, and wheelchairs. When our bodies slow down to the point that we cannot take care of ourselves anymore, doctors call it "functional decline." The essential functions that we do every day are often taken for granted.

Think of all the things we do to get up in the morning and get out the door: wake up, sit up in bed, stand up from bed, walk to the bathroom, toilet and wipe, brush our teeth, take a shower, get dressed, feed ourselves breakfast, and walk out the door. These are called "ADLs" or activities of daily living. If we cannot independently do these ADLs, we die—unless we can hire someone to do it for us.

When we lose our ability to do our ADLs and our organ functions slow down, we may get admitted to the hospital more frequently and not improve much despite rehabilitation. It's like an old boat or automobile, the parts start to fail: the engine, the brakes, the transmission, the battery, etc. You can fix it here and there and take it to the shop multiple times, but the vehicle is dying anyway. This is when the end-of-life cycle starts.

WHEN IT'S YOUR STOP, YOU GOT TO GET OFF

My brother had many losses, including three friends from his group home, his high school teacher, and his neighbor/friend. Several of them died one after the other, during the COVID pandemic, and Peter could not make sense of this. He became depressed, ate less, lost weight, withdrew more, and began to stay in his room. My parents and I became concerned, and so did his doctor.

After doing some medical work up, we all realized that Peter did not have a physical problem. He was grieving. Grief and depression often look similar, and it takes some time to untangle. After a while, my mom sat down to talk to him. She told Peter, "You know how you take the subway, and you have to know your stop. When it's your stop, you gotta get off. That's what happened to your friends and teacher. Life is like a train. When it's your stop, you gotta get off."

It was like a lightbulb went off in his head. He called me up and said, "I know what happened to my teacher and my friends. It was their stop. And they had to get off. There's nothing they could do about it." He was at peace.

LESSONS

- Look at end of life as part of the life cycle and part of your journey. If we're lucky, we will get there some day. In the meantime, enjoy the ride!
- Learn as much as you can about palliative care and hospice. Attend local talks, request your local hospital to make a presentation for the community, and look for resources online. Doing this type of homework will help you better prepare for serious illness and end of life.
- Embrace your emotions—both laughter and tears. Let the emotions come over you! Happiness and sadness are reflections of a full, rich life. Have you considered this: if you feel pain or sadness, that means you are alive! And that is precious.

APPENDIX

Additional Resources

There are many additional resources I've come across that I wanted to share with you. Maybe they can help you as you consider advance directives for you and your loved ones.

NATIONAL INSTITUTE ON AGING

The National Institute on Aging compiled a list of advance care planning tips that I wholeheartedly support:[17]

- Reflect on your values and wishes.
- Talk with your doctor about advance directives.
- Choose someone you trust to make medical decisions for you.

---

17 "Advance Care Planning: Advance Directives for Health Care," National Institute on Aging, October 31, 2022, https://www.nia.nih.gov/health/advance-care-planning/advance-care-planning-advance-directives-health-care.

- Complete your advance directive forms.
- Share your forms with your healthcare proxy, doctors, and loved ones.
- Keep the conversation going.

THE CONVERSATION PROJECT

The Conversation Project, part of the IHI (Institute for Healthcare Improvement)[18] has an entire website devoted to advance directives and end-of-life planning. That website includes a 12-page guide that taps into someone's wishes and dreams for the rest of their life and approaches advance directives in a warm and welcoming way. One of the key questions is, "What matters to me through the end of my life is ..."

THE STANFORD LETTER PROJECT

The Stanford Letter Project (https://med.stanford.edu/letter.html) contains form letters that you can

---

18 "The Conversation Project," Institute for Healthcare Improvement, accessed January 23, 2024, https://theconversationproject.org/.

address to your friends and family and your primary care physician, allowing people to identify what matters most to them as they face end-of-life care.

FIVE WISHES

Five Wishes aims to document someone's wishes for their healthcare proxy, their treatment choices, their comfort level, how they want to be treated, and what they want their loved ones to know. Notably, Five Wishes comes in multiple languages and is accepted in a majority of states.

PREPARE FOR YOUR CARE

Prepare for Your Care (https://prepareforyourcare.org/en/welcome) has a step-by-step program with video examples for your care and the care for others.

GET PALLIATIVE CARE

Get Palliative Care (https://getpalliativecare.org/) features information and handouts to help you and your family navigate serious illness. It also features stories of others receiving palliative care to help you recognize that others are facing similar circumstances.

THE DEATH OF IVAN ILYICH

Leo Tolstoy's *The Death of Ivan Ilyich* tells the story of a high-court judge in 19th-century Russia and his sufferings and death from a terminal illness. During the long and painful process of dying, Ivan believed he did not deserve his suffering because he had lived rightly. Ivan began to hate his family for avoiding the subject of his death and for pretending he is only sick and not dying. He found his only comfort in his peasant boy servant, Gerasim, the only person who did not fear death and showed compassion for him. Ivan began to question whether he had, in fact, lived a good life.

Additional Resources

THE 36-HOUR DAY: A FAMILY GUIDE TO CARING FOR PEOPLE WHO HAVE ALZHEIMER DISEASE AND OTHER DEMENTIAS

Written by Nancy L. Mace, MA, and Peter V. Rabins, MD, MPH, *The 36-Hour Day*[19] has been the leading work in the field for caregivers of those with dementia. The authors have decades of experience caring for individuals with memory loss, Alzheimer's, and other dementias. The book is widely known for its comprehensive information and compassionate approach to care.

THE FOUR THINGS THAT MATTER MOST

Dr. Ira Byock's *The Four Things That Matter Most: A Book About Living*[20] deals with four simple phrases—Please forgive me, I forgive you, thank you, and I love you—and we encourage family members and patients to make peace by using these phrases. Simple sayings

---

19 Nancy L. Mace and Peter V. Rabins, *The 36-Hour Day*, 7th ed. (Baltimore, MD: Johns Hopkins University Press, 2021).
20 Ira Byock, *The Four Things That Matter Most*, 10th-anniversary edition (New York: Atria Books, 2014).

like those, and "I'm going to be okay," can give patients the permission to move forward on their journey.

CAN'T WE TALK ABOUT SOMETHING MORE PLEASANT?

The book *Can't We Talk About Something More Pleasant?* by Roz Chast, a longtime *New Yorker* cartoonist, details her parents' final years in heartfelt but darkly humorous fashion. The cover—showing her sitting down with her frustrated parents—perfectly captures the mood of discussing advance directives.[21]

THE TOOLS

The Tools: 5 Tools to Help You Find Courage, Creativity, and Willpower—and Inspire You to Live Life in Forward Motion by Phil Stutz and Barry Michels is a self-help book that provides practical tools to confront and overcome fear, pain, and other emotional

---

21 Chast, *Can't We Talk About Something More Pleasant?*

Additional Resources

obstacles.[22] It offers a new perspective on life, helping readers to thrive and live in the present moment. This applies to end-of-life care beautifully. As an example, Dr. Stutz's book involves a mental exercise that can help you face the pain ("Bring it on!"), move toward the pain ("I love pain!"), and find freedom ("Pain sets me free!").

---

22 Phil Stutz and Barry Michels, *The Tools: 5 Tools to Help You Find Courage, Creativity, and Willpower—and Inspire You to Live Life in Forward Motion* (New York: Random House, 2023).

Acknowledgments

Working in palliative care and hospice settings, I always like to say, "Teamwork makes the dream work!" I have many people to thank who supported me through the many years it took to make this book happen. I will express my gratitude and appreciation team by team.

MY FAMILY TEAM

- Hsiang—my mom! You are an angel, a saint, the most patient and nonjudgmental human being ever. You inspire me with your support, wise emails, and inspirational WeChat messages. You give the best hugs and feed us all amazing food filled with love.
- James—my dad! A visionary who brought us to America and gave us so many

opportunities, opening the doors for us. You wrote and published and inspired me to follow in your footsteps. You were stern, and now you express love and appreciation for us. You passed away in April 2024, and we miss you dearly. I later found a note you wrote in support of my book. I will treasure it!

- Darrell—my dear husband who knows me, finishes my sentences, and reads my mind sometimes. You support and encourage me on my book writing and publishing journey. When I showed you a selfie I took at an airport book stand, you texted me, "You will get there!" Thank you for giving me advice and feedback about my book title and cover design ideas, and thank you for your unwavering support. You told me to be "The Dr. Ruth of Palliative Care"! ☺
- Christopher—my son! You write me the best notes and cards with personal messages—a lost art, when you think about it. You always remember to get or make me a gift for my birthday, Mother's Day, Christmas. You

Acknowledgments

surprise me with texts and videos appreciating me as your mom. I appreciate you!

- CJ—my son! You call me "ma" in the most affectionate way! You show your loving support by running errands and driving our families for get-togethers. You always share things that bring you joy, like your song list, memes, and what you think are funny jokes. JK!
- Peter—my little brother! You call me "Number One" because I'm the oldest. Even though you were born with developmental disabilities and cannot read or write or do math, you have a beautiful spirit and social network. Even though you can't work or make money, you sent me your saved-up money when we ran into hard times and I was worried about my mortgage payments. You call me every week to remind me to watch our mutual favorite show on Food Network, *Restaurant: Impossible*, and to tell me about the weather. ☺
- Kai—my middle brother! You taught me so much about personal finance and supported me in accounting for my finances!

Exit Strategies

After the COVID pandemic, you saw that I was working very hard and had accumulated take-out food containers, so you brought me cooking resources—an air fryer oven, sous vide immersion cooker, flavoring packets and sauces—and taught me to cook good food efficiently. When you come visit and stay with me for a weekend, I always wake up to amazing aromas: fresh coffee, pancakes, Vietnamese noodles, pork roast, cookies, and more. You rock!

- Irene—my mom-in-law, bless your soul. You were kind, even if we disagreed sometimes. Thank you for always thinking of me and buying me clothes and shoes that I would not get for myself. You have a great eye, and you know so much about so many topics. You always treated me like a daughter, and I appreciate that! I wish you were here!
- Gerry—my beautiful and witty aunt-in-law! Thank you for reading my draft chapters and encouraging me to keep going.
- Clara—my beautiful and wise aunt! Thank you for reading my early work, giving me

Acknowledgments

advice and feedback, asking me about the book, and keeping me accountable.
- Susan—my beautiful and high-spirited cousin! You have the best laughter in the whole world. You send me cookies and treats to keep me going. You always gave my parents rides to get-togethers. Even my dad began to ask, whenever we had an event, "Is Susan coming?"
- Shannon—my sis! You always call or text to check how I'm doing. Even when you were not well, you were thinking of me and keeping me going! You have a beautiful heart.
- Melina—my niece! Thank you for asking me about my book progress and showing interest, and for asking for a signed copy! You motivated me to start building my "book army" list!
- Jie, Chloe, and Liam—thank you for your warm support and for putting my presale date in your calendars! I'm counting on you! ☺
- Gary and Kim—thank you for believing in me!

MY FRIENDS TEAM

- Lisa Katzman—my best friend from high school! I truly appreciate our precious friendship. You are always willing to help out even when I don't ask. So full of heart. Thank you for reintroducing me to Broadway shows and for always being available to talk through my book challenges!
- Joyce, Esther, Alex, and Cheryl, my Great Neck "Joy Luck Club"! Thank you for asking about my book and how I am doing. I look forward to our monthly get-togethers and check-ins with each other!
- Jason and Ella—thank you for checking in and asking me about the progress of my book. I truly needed accountability!
- Sunitha Polepalle—you came back into my life during COVID, when I was out of breath and scared. I am thankful you introduced me to the Art of Living team, who helped me meditate and breathe again!

Acknowledgments

- Calvin Hwang—I treasure our walks and talks together. Thank you for giving me the tip to prone myself when I was sick with COVID!
- Maria Lee—you are always here to support me. Thank you for your advice and encouragement!
- Marta Kazandjian—you are my soul sister! Thank you for your positive spirit and for being a role model for writing books!
- My Harvard alum friends and the H4A! Even with the distance and our busy schedules, I know I can always come home to this community!

MY COLLEAGUES TEAM

- Diane Meier—my mentor, who helped me without hesitation! You taught me to have high clinical standards and trust my medical judgment. You were the first one to read my ARC and endorse my book. I'm forever thankful!

- Sean Morrison—you inspired me to write up my research results and set high bars for clinical excellence.
- Jane Morris—thank you for your wisdom and friendship and advocacy. Love our late afternoon coffee runs and dinners together at Chef Wang. If it were not for you, I would not have a favorite Chinese restaurant that now routinely gives us a discount if we pay cash. Thank you Stephanie for your encouragement and for teaching me how to make the best pizza ever!
- Fernando Kawai—we mentor and inspire each other. We always joked that we are connected in a karmic way. You're Japanese and Brazilian. I'm Chinese with Latina blood from growing up all over South America. Your spirit keeps me going and supports me. Thank you Julienne for your warmth, support, and smiles!
- Rosanne Leipzig—you helped me with one of my first papers, spending time and money doing phone conferences even though you

Acknowledgments

were away for a conference. Thank you for your generosity!

- Jennie Chin-Hansen—you always inspire me with your leadership, kindness, and advocacy! Thank you for reading my book and for all your feedback!
- Matthew Castillo—you are loyal, kind, supportive, and humorous, and you check in on all of us. You always know when to bring me a surprise cappuccino when I need it most. Even though I mentor you, you have taught me so much about psychological safety and teamwork! You are the best!
- My amazing NewYork-Presbyterian Queens (NYPQ) palliative care and geriatrics team—Robert Crupi, Matthew Castillo, Dhrity Bhowmik, Benjamin Fay, Latrice Pelissier, Hoda Abdelaziz, Latoya Duckett, Michelle Solat, Wing Fun Leo-To, Elizabeth Schlesinger, and Sandra Cardenas-Arroyave! Also my bosses and mentors, Amir Jaffer and Joseph Cooke, who are both inspirations to me. And my fabulous GME team, especially Janet Ramirez!

- Colleagues at Hospice Care Network—Maureen Hinkelman, Tanveer Mir, Lori Attivissimo, Eirene Milano, Tara Liberman, Nan Toelstedt, Jane Morris, Amy Resnick, Sue Sturgess, and many more—you gave me the opportunity and honor to care for remarkable hospice patients. We had good times sharing much-needed massages and sushi after tough days.
- Chinese American Medical Society (CAMS) colleagues—Victor Chang, Warren Chin, Mary Lee-Wong, Benjamin Lee, Jamie Love, Joanna Li, Gomeo Lam, Cora Fung, Alex Ky, Ning Lin, Paul Lee, James Tsai, Yick Moon Lee, and the whole team—I learned so much from you, working together on scientific programming, leadership, and wellness and speaking up for the Chinese and Asian American communities.
- Chinese American Nurses Association (CANA) colleagues, especially Theresa Chan! Thank you for your support, community work, and willingness to help promote my book!

Acknowledgments

- Chinese American IPA (CAIPA) colleagues, especially Peggy Shen! Thank you for teaching me about advocacy for our communities!
- Visiting Nurse Service (VNS) Health colleagues, especially Ritchell Dignam and Teresa Lin! Thank you for your eternal support, for promoting interdisciplinary and fellowship education, and for supporting my book writing journey.
- Metropolitan Jewish Health System (MJHS) Hospice colleagues, especially Toby Weiss, Kerriann Page, our NYPQ liaisons Princess and Bithia, and many more!
- Eric Widera—you inspire me with your sensibility and can-do attitude, plus your rock star podcast, *GeriPal*!
- Chinese American Coalition for Compassionate Care (CACCC) colleagues, especially Sandy Chen-Stokes and Shirley Pan—what a team!

MY ACCOUNTABILITY TEAM

- The Book Launchers team—Roy, Renee, Kate, and Dan Good, just to name a few! And of course Julie and Angela. What an amazing team! I'm so lucky I found you!
- Maria Corvese—my well-being coach! You are one of my early accountability partners for this book! Thank you.
- Gail Gazelle—my physician coach. Thank you so much for helping me find the "new me," face and conquer my fears (most of them, anyway), and build my "inner ally" and "observer role." I treasure our talks together.

This is an overwhelming and very emotional time for me. I may have missed some people in my acknowledgments. I send you warm air hugs and all my best wishes in advance!

Notes

www.ingramcontent.com/pod-product-compliance
Lightning Source LLC
LaVergne TN
LVHW091531070526
838199LV00001B/23